The Low-Cholesterol Cookbook & Health Plan

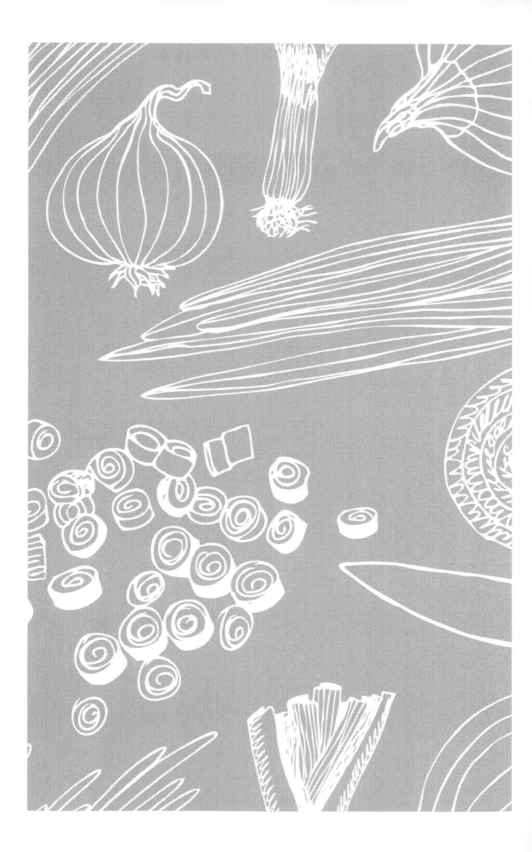

The Low-Cholesterol Cookbook & Health Plan

MEAL PLANS AND LOW-FAT RECIPES *to* IMPROVE HEART HEALTH

SHASTA PRESS

Contents

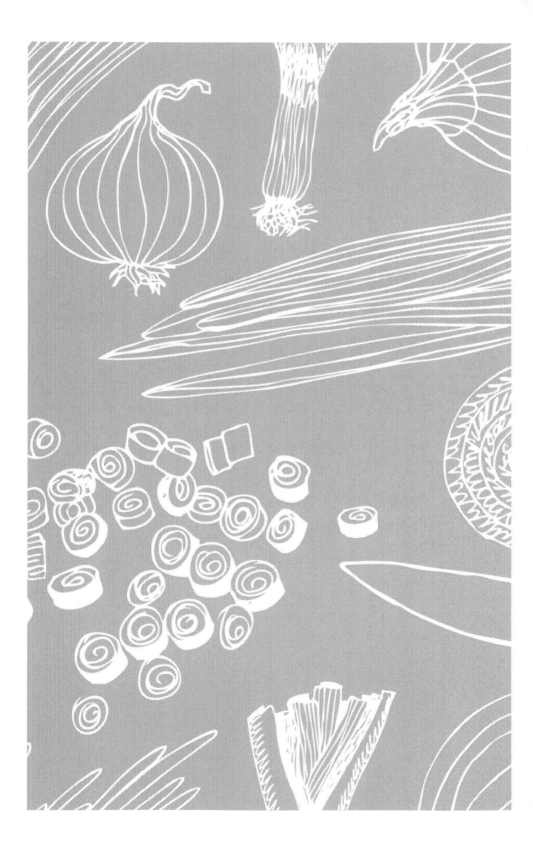

Introduction

Many people agree that maintaining the right amounts of cholesterol can be key to heart health, but if you are unsure what to eat to keep your cholesterol in balance or are even confused about what cholesterol is, you are not alone. Although much maligned, this waxy substance is needed—in the right proportion—to create hormones and vitamins as well as to help you digest food. And it keeps your cells and nerves healthy and intact.

Even when cholesterol collects in your arteries, research now shows that it is there to cover and compensate for damage that can sometimes occur to your artery walls. Problems may arise, however, when too much cholesterol collects in the bloodstream and obstructs passageways that lead to your heart and brain. While nobody would intentionally clog their own arteries, it's possible to do just that with the food choices that you make. Ordering fast food on a time-crunched schedule, grabbing a sweet treat to boost energy, or equating comfort food with only fat-laden meat-and-potatoes meals are behaviors that can raise unhealthful cholesterol levels.

If you think that more people die from a broken heart than any other ailment, you are essentially correct. Heart disease is the leading cause of death in North Americans over the age of forty-five, and high cholesterol is one of the known risk factors. One in six adults, or 17 percent of the U.S. population, has high cholesterol. According to the Centers for Disease Control and Prevention (CDC), people with high cholesterol have twice the risk of heart disease as people with normal levels.

While these numbers can be alarming, if you have been told that you need to lower your cholesterol—or if you're just trying to eat healthier—this book will help you take a few basic steps to achieve or maintain low cholesterol and keep it at a healthful level for life. It will also answer your questions about this complex and often baffling substance in practical, easy-to-understand terms. You'll feel confident to tackle cholesterol-related health issues head-on, especially once you discover the tempting array of tasty cholesterol-lowering appetizers, side dishes, entrées, and desserts.

THE 1 + 1 – 1 EATING PLAN

The low-cholesterol diet presented in this book uses a simple addition and subtraction method to help you control your cholesterol numbers. The 1 + 1 – 1 Eating Plan works like this:

- *Add* foods that are low in cholesterol.
- *Add* foods that increase good cholesterol and decrease inflammation.
- *Subtract* foods that are high in cholesterol and that increase bad cholesterol.

The recipes that accompany the 1 + 1 – 1 Eating Plan include nutritional information to help you plan balanced meals as well as keep track of your cholesterol intake. When you make conscious rather than habitual eating choices, your cholesterol levels will fall. Not only will your blood flow more freely through your arteries, you will also likely feel more healthy, vital, and inclined to be more active.

LOOK WHAT'S INSIDE

With more than one hundred easy-to-make recipes, this go-to guide offers a practical eating program that's simple to incorporate into your lifestyle. Chapter One includes an explanation of the science behind your cholesterol numbers and introduces you to the 1 + 1 – 1 Eating Plan, the backbone of the many flavorful and nutritious recipes in this book designed to help you achieve and maintain healthful cholesterol levels. Chapter Two offers specific guidelines for the 1 + 1 – 1 Eating Plan, including certain foods whose nutrients raise good cholesterol levels, as well as foods to avoid or reduce in your diet to help lower cholesterol.

Lifestyle changes to help lower cholesterol, tips on making smart restaurant choices, dietary considerations if you are taking cholesterol medication, and handy substitutions and alternatives for cooking and baking are covered in Chapter Three. In Chapter Four you'll find a fourteen-day meal plan that you can use as a guide to create your own menus.

The recipe chapters that follow are organized by meal type and offer a variety of easy, cholesterol-lowering recipes that contain nutrients your body needs. Low in cholesterol as well as processed and saturated fats, these recipes have little to no sugar, processed flour, or salt. They feature lean proteins, fiber-rich vegetables, and filling whole grains. They include healthful fish recipes for omega-3s; whole-grain pasta and pasta alternatives for fiber; quick stir-fries loaded with crisp, nutrient-rich vegetables; and comfort-food breakfasts that use sly substitutions to help lower your cholesterol. Plus, most of these truly mouthwatering recipes can be prepared in thirty minutes or less!

Whether your goal is to lower your cholesterol or simply maintain overall good health, you can enjoy the benefits of the 1 + 1 – 1 Eating Plan as part of your personal routine. Try the low-cholesterol meal strategies and lifestyle suggestions, and celebrate healthful results as you follow this book's credo: Healthful choices don't have to be flavorless choices.

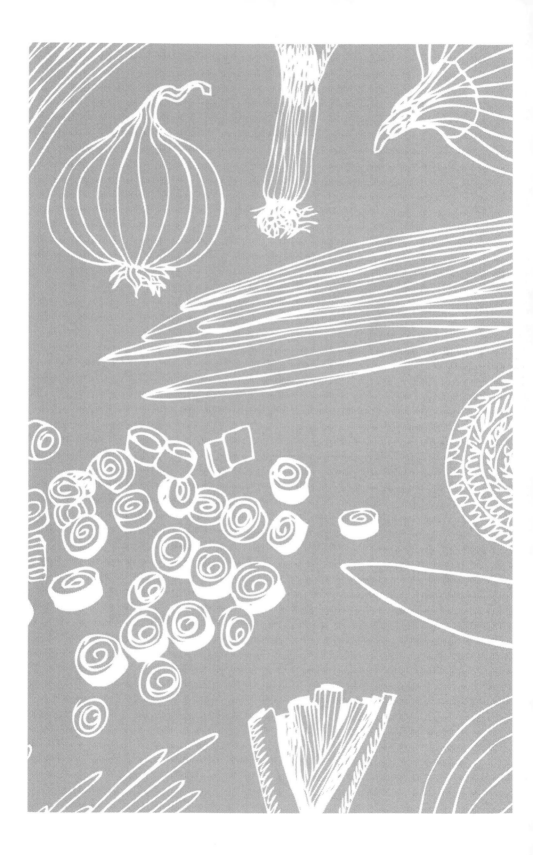

PART ONE

The Low-Cholesterol Diet

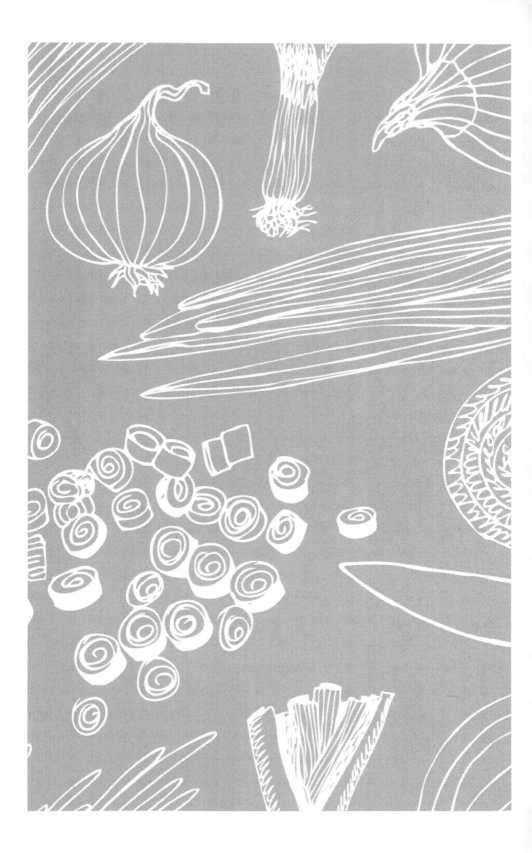

CHAPTER ONE

What Is the Low-Cholesterol Diet?

If your cholesterol numbers are too high—or too low—it can seem like an arduous task to nudge those numbers in the right direction. Although cholesterol is vital for your body to function, the key is balance—having just the right amounts of both low-density lipoprotein (LDL) and high-density lipoprotein (HDL) cholesterol.

Current National Cholesterol Education Program guidelines say your body's total cholesterol should be no more than 200 mg/dL (mg per deciliter of blood), which breaks down to 100 mg/dL or less LDL (often termed "bad" cholesterol) and 40 mg/dL or higher HDL ("good" cholesterol). Although a default method for lowering bad cholesterol is using medication, research shows that certain nutrients in foods, when working in combination, can be as powerful as medicine. While taking a little longer, natural methods help lower heart disease and stroke risk without some of the negative side effects associated with medications. If you are already taking cholesterol-lowering medication, the dietary changes recommended here can enhance its effectiveness.

With a few simple lifestyle and diet adjustments to help set you on the right course, *The Low-Cholesterol Cookbook & Health Plan* guides you with a simple 1 + 1 – 1 Eating Plan to keep your cholesterol numbers in check. Meanwhile, you will enjoy getting back to the basics of real, fresh whole food in all its delightful colors, aromas, and pure tastes. The recipes in this book feature everyday "superhero" foods known to help raise good HDL cholesterol. When eaten alone, these foods have a positive impact, but when eaten together, they unite in a powerful cholesterol-lowering boost that rivals medication and provides a symphony of fresh flavors.

WHAT IS CHOLESTEROL?

Cholesterol is a waxy, fat-like substance found in your body and in many foods. While the media may have bombarded you with the belief that all cholesterol is bad, the opposite is true. Your body requires cholesterol for many important functions: It is vital in making hormones like testosterone, estrogen, and progesterone; it makes digestive acids (commonly called bile); and it is used in the myelin sheath covering your nerves. You get approximately 90 percent of the body's daily cholesterol requirement from your liver, and 10 percent is obtained from diet.

The liver makes cholesterol, and the intestines absorb cholesterol from food and digestive acids. For some people, the liver produces more cholesterol than the intestines can absorb. Others end up with too much cholesterol because of lifestyle factors, including the foods they eat, the amount of activity they get, and the rate at which their bodies break down cholesterol. A healthful diet and regular exercise can help balance your cholesterol levels and improve your cardiovascular system, which includes the heart and blood vessels that carry nutrients and oxygen to the rest of your body.

"Good" versus "Bad" Cholesterol

Low-density lipoprotein (LDL) is a very fatty protein. A lipoprotein with more fat and less protein is less dense; therefore, it is more apt to mix with your blood to make it have a high fat content. LDL makes up most of the body's cholesterol, and is often called "bad" because high levels—especially of a type of LDL called Lp(a)—may lead to heart disease and stroke. However, your body needs a certain level of LDL to sustain itself, so LDL is really only bad when it's out of balance.

- -

Lp(a) or lipoprotein(a) is a genetic variation of bad cholesterol. A high level of Lp(a) may interact with substances found in artery walls to make fatty deposits build up.

- -

High-density lipoprotein, or dense fatty protein, is called "good" cholesterol because high levels may reduce the risk of heart disease and stroke. Scientists think that HDL absorbs bad cholesterol and carries it to the liver, which then flushes it from the body.

The Inside Story: Your Arteries

To imagine what the inside of your arteries look like, picture a long pipe with an outer wall and a few layers of inner lining made of skin-like tissue and smooth muscle. Within this "pipe," blood is carried at a brisk pace throughout your body. Problems can occur when a layer of plaque—composed of cholesterol, triglycerides (a type of fat), heavy metals (toxins), collagen, and waste held together by calcium—collects and builds up in your pipe-like arteries. Over time, this plaque narrows your artery passages, blocking the blood's route to your heart, brain, and other organs. Plaque can also break off and travel, creating blood clots that cause damage elsewhere in your system. Simple blood tests can be done to check cholesterol levels in your blood and determine if your arteries may be at risk for developing plaque, which can lead to heart disease (also called atherosclerosis).

The *Route* of the Problem

Having a lot of cholesterol-coated plaque is actually a symptom of something else going on beneath the plaque on the arteries themselves. Two-time Nobel Prize winner Dr. Linus Pauling discovered that this cholesterol-laden plaque is in fact trying to protect you. The process begins when nicks and tears are created along the arterial wall by tiny tumors that have burst. Such tumors are attributable to poor lifestyle choices leading to chronic inflammation, as well as chemical irritants (such as nicotine) and diseases like diabetes. The body's clotting fiber moves in to patch the tear, and it's this protective fiber that ends up trapping cholesterol, calcium, fats, and other substances.

Plaque buildup can take many years to develop, but waiting for symptoms to surface is a bad idea. There are no symptoms for high cholesterol, and heart disease is called the "silent killer" for its lack of obvious signs. Yet plaque buildup and cholesterol imbalance are preventable and treatable with simple changes in lifestyle and eating habits. A few changes you can make right now will pay off in the future.

Simplifying the Cholesterol Equation

Cholesterol is found in every cell of the body and is a cell protector, which is good. It becomes worrisome only when too much of it is found in two specific areas: your blood and your artery walls. *The Low-Cholesterol Cookbook & Health Plan* specifically addresses both of these concerns.

THE LOW-CHOLESTEROL DIET

The Low-Cholesterol Cookbook & Health Plan uses a simple addition and sub-traction approach to help you control your cholesterol numbers and keep your arterial passageways clear, healthy, and strong. It lets you choose foods that help reduce the formation of miniscule tears that cause cholesterol to cling to your vulnerable arteries. *The Low-Cholesterol Cookbook & Health Plan* 1 + 1 – 1 Eating Plan has three key components easily translated into the meals you eat throughout the day. Whether you're preparing meals at home or dining out, once you understand the guidelines and which of your favorite foods to choose, you can incorporate this handy method into your daily routine and watch your results multiply.

The following pages outline the 1 + 1 – 1 Eating Plan in three easy steps:

- *Add* foods that are low in cholesterol.
- *Add* foods that increase good cholesterol and decrease inflammation.
- *Subtract* foods that are high in cholesterol and that increase bad cholesterol.

Add Foods That Are Low in Cholesterol

Foods that come from plants have no cholesterol. That means all vegetables, fruits, legumes, seeds, nuts, and whole, unprocessed grains are in high demand on the low-cholesterol diet. Although the United States Department of Agri-culture (USDA) recommends seven servings of vegetables and one serving of fruit daily, these are minimum requirements. The 1 + 1 – 1 Eating Plan recom-mends eight to ten servings of vegetables and two servings of fruit each day. These numbers are not difficult to achieve, especially when you combine sev-eral types of vegetables in one dish, such as in a salad, stir-fry, or pasta sauce, or in a casserole or stew in which vegetables are the star attraction. Also, the size of one serving (such as a half cup of cooked vegetables) as outlined in the USDA's Food Guide is not large. See page 19 for more on serving portions.

Vegetables and fruits vary in fat content, but most of the fat found in these foods is monounsaturated or polyunsaturated fat—in other words, healthful fats that you need to combat cholesterol. For example, apples, oranges, melons, leafy greens, carrots, potatoes, and celery contain almost no fat, and avocados, olives, seeds, nuts, and coconut have a high good-fat content.

Add Foods That Increase Good Cholesterol and Decrease Inflammation

Some everyday foods act like superheroes to stave off bad cholesterol and fortify and heal your arteries. A diet including the right amounts of good fats, fiber, vitamins, and minerals will help balance your cholesterol and protect against inflammation.

Good Fats: Omega-3 fatty acids are unsaturated fats effective in balancing cholesterol and protecting against inflammation that can cause tears in artery walls. A 2004 study in the *Archives of Internal Medicine* found that omega-3 fish oils were even more protective than cholesterol-lowering drugs. A type of omega-3 fat called alpha-linolenic acid (ALA) is found in nuts, seeds, and some vegetables; the omega-3 fats eicosapentaenoic acid (EPA) and docosahexaenoic acid (DHA) are found in fatty fish.

The American Heart Association's diet and lifestyle recommendations advise people to consume fish, especially oily fish, at least twice a week, stating: "The consumption of 8 ounces per week of fish high in EPA and DHA is associated with a reduced risk of coronary artery disease in adults."

Omega-6 and omega-9 fatty acids, found in vegetables and seed oils, also help lower bad cholesterol and reduce inflammation.

According to the USDA, your total fat intake should be between 20 and 35 percent of your total daily calories, with most fats coming from sources of polyunsaturated and monounsaturated fatty acids such as fish, nuts, and seed oils. See page 14 for a list of foods that contain good fats.

Fiber: Eating more fibrous vegetables has been shown to have dramatic effects on blood cholesterol levels. A Harvard University study, for example, found that people who consumed eight or more servings of fruits and vegetables a day had a 20 percent lower risk of heart disease than those who ate fewer than three servings. Part of that result is believed to be related to fiber content and the role it plays in cholesterol reduction.

Insoluble fiber attaches itself to the fat from food and cholesterol in the gut and takes it out of your body in your stool—so the fat isn't absorbed by the body. Insoluble fiber is found in the skins of vegetables and fruit, and in the bran of whole grains.

Soluble fiber helps slow the absorption of cholesterol and reduce the amount of cholesterol the liver makes. When water is added to soluble fiber, it thickens and becomes sticky and gel-like. Soluble fiber can be found in some vegetables, fruit, and seeds, and in some types of bran and legumes.

See page 15 for information about fruits, vegetables, seeds, and grains that are high in health-giving fiber.

Whole, unprocessed plant-derived foods contain powerful, protecting nutrients, including antioxidant vitamins C and E, vitamin B, and certain minerals, which help to balance cholesterol and protect against damage that can lead to artery nicks and tears.

Vitamin C: Vitamin C helps to raise HDL (good) and lower LDL (bad) cholesterol, keeps blood vessels flexible, reduces plaque formation, and vitamin C also makes collagen, which is vital for the repair and regeneration of your arteries. Vitamin C is found in berries, fruits, and some vegetables.

. . . .

The National Health and Nutrition Examination Survey (NHANES) showed the risk of death from cardiovascular diseases was 42 percent lower in men and 25 percent lower in women who consumed more than 50 mg per day of dietary vitamin C.

. . . .

Vitamin E: Vitamin E promotes cardiovascular function and reduces "inflammatory markers," which include cholesterol levels. The largest study on vitamin E and heart health to date, part of the Harvard-based Nurses' Health Study and Health Professionals Follow-up Study, involving 39,876 women over the age of forty-five, found that vitamin E significantly reduced the number of heart disease–related deaths. Vitamin E is found in greens, seeds, and nuts.

Vitamin B Complex: Vitamin B complex includes niacin, folic acid, choline, and inositol, all of which are very important to your health. Niacin (vitamin B3) enlarges blood vessels, helps to eliminate excess cholesterol, and metabolizes fats. Folic acid may substantially reduce the incidence of cardiovascular disease. Choline prevents fat from sticking to arteries, and inositol is a relaxant;

low levels of choline and inositol trigger high cholesterol. These B vitamins are found in whole, unprocessed grains, and in certain vegetables and meat.

Minerals: Certain minerals are also vital. Necessary for many areas of heart health, magnesium keeps calcium and cholesterol from sticking to artery walls. It's in nuts and in dark, leafy greens. Potassium, found in seeds and fruits, helps regulate blood pressure levels. Selenium, found in grains and seeds, may help lower total cholesterol levels. Other nutrients that may help reduce cholesterol include curcumin, found in the spice turmeric; lutein, found in greens; sulfur, found in garlic; sterols and stanols, found in grains and some vegetables; and antioxidant flavonoids, found in dark chocolate.

Subtract Foods That Are High in Cholesterol and That Increase Bad Cholesterol

What the foods you eat do not have is as important as what they do have. To help decrease cholesterol and inflammation, reduce certain fats, processed foods, and sugar.

Trans fats: Avoid trans fats, which are vegetable oils that have been chemically manipulated or "hydrogenated" to become dense and hardened (to look and act like saturated fats, such as lard and butter, which are more expensive to use). Trans fats are not found in nature, and the human body has difficulty absorbing and using them. Trans fats lower good HDL cholesterol and raise bad LDL cholesterol—the opposite of what you need. The USDA recommends not eating them at all.

Saturated fats: Saturated fat isn't all bad (and some types, like what is found in coconut, are thought to be good for you), but too much animal fat increases blood fat and cholesterol levels. Saturated fats are found in animal products, including poultry, seafood, dairy, eggs, and even the leanest meats. When selecting animal protein, make choices that are lean or low-fat to limit saturated amounts. One food to eat sparingly is shrimp, which doesn't have much fat but has twice the cholesterol of beef or chicken.

. . . .

According to the USDA, less than 10 percent of calories consumed in a day should come from saturated fats.

. . . .

Full-fat dairy products are the main sources of saturated fat in many people's diets. Saturated fat is also hidden in store-bought baked goods and in processed foods (foods that no longer look like they did in nature). In addition to cutting back on fatty meats, the Food and Drug Administration (FDA) stipulates dramatically reducing whole milk, fatty cheeses, butter, margarine, processed oils, lard, cream, egg yolks, fried foods, and fatty desserts. These are high in cholesterol in addition to saturated fat.

Reduce Omega-6 Fats Found in Processed Oils. Omega-6 fats are found in vegetable oils, including margarine, and in cooking oils, such as sunflower, safflower, cottonseed, and canola oil. Although you need omega-6 in your diet, too much creates inflammation in the body. Science has shown that the ratio of omega-6 to omega-3 fats in a healthful diet should be about 1:1, and no more than 5:1, a ratio found naturally in many foods such as seeds, nuts, and unrefined vegetable oils. If you eat many processed foods with added cooking oils, you may regularly consume a ratio of as much as 20:1. In that case, you need to increase your omega-3 intake while decreasing consumption of processed omega-6 oils. The recipes in this book call for very sparing use of oils that have been highly processed.

Avoid Simple Carbohydrates and Sugar. The amount of simple carbohydrates and sugars you eat can sneak up unnoticed. According to the USDA, added sugars should comprise no more than 25 percent of the total calories you eat in a day. "Added sugars" are not those that occur naturally, such as in whole fruit, but those that are added during manufacturing in processed foods; added sugars also include those found in baked goods, both purchased and homemade. Although major sources of added sugars include soft drinks, fruit juices, desserts, and sweets, you will find sugar listed on the back of almost all canned and boxed foods, usually added to improve the flavor and entice you to eat more of that food.

White wheat flour and white rice are devoid of most nutrients, because the germ and bran of these grains has been removed to enable them to be stored for a long time without spoiling. Like sugar, too much of these nutrient-poor foods causes inflammation and triggers harmful LDL cholesterol. In a review of more than two hundred studies, researchers linked eating high-glycemic-index (GI) foods such as sugar, white rice, and white bread with increased cardiovascular risk.

Buy and prepare your foods and beverages with little added sugars or chemical (artificial) sweeteners. Instead, use more healthful sweeteners in limited amounts. And switch to whole grains, such as those suggested by the USDA. This doesn't mean you can't enjoy desserts and treats. It simply means replacing certain flours and sweeteners for others that taste as good. See pages 25 and 26 for the best flours and sweeteners to use.

Subtract Salt. Avoid sodium chloride, meaning regular table salt, in cooking and in packaged products. Instead, use natural substitutes. Any word that includes "sodium" on an ingredient list is salt. According to Health Canada, the average adult consumes over 3,100 mg of sodium each day. Reduce this unhealthful number to between 1,200 and 1,500 mg of sodium daily, as recommended by Health Canada and the U.S. National Academy of Sciences, Institute of Medicine.

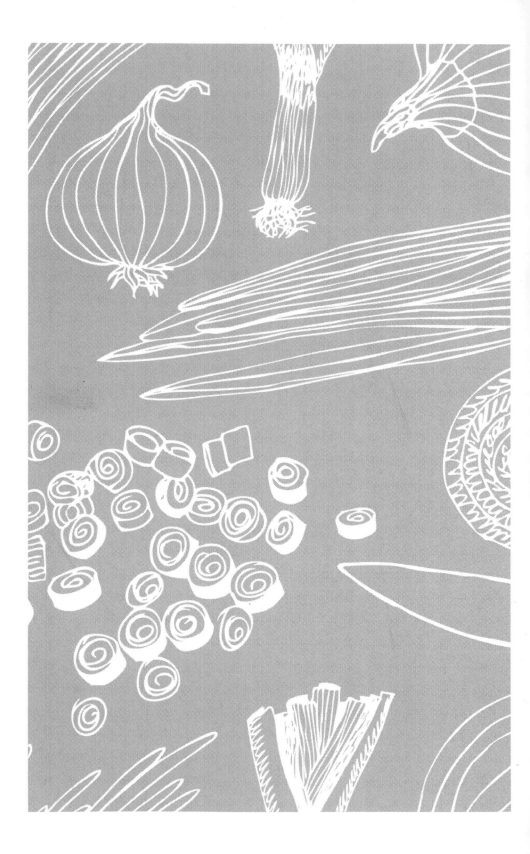

CHAPTER TWO

Getting Started on the Low-Cholesterol Diet

When Bruce Springsteen sings, "Everybody's got a hungry heart," you know he's not referring to food, but everybody does have a heart hungry for certain nutrients that will keep it healthy for a lifetime. From oats to spinach to walnuts, everyday foods are stepping up to the plate when it comes to controlling cholesterol. *The Low-Cholesterol Cookbook & Health Plan* 1 + 1 – 1 Eating Plan encourages you to make healthier choices by understanding which foods raise good cholesterol levels, and which foods to reduce or avoid in your diet. For starters, cook up some color. Vibrant greens in salads, bold oranges in curries, full-bodied reds in tomato sauce, and sunny yellows in citrus fruit can all positively affect impact your cholesterol. By learning to decipher food labels, consciously considering each meal's ingredients, and serving appropriate portions, you can begin to balance your cholesterol—and feed your hungry heart.

LOW-CHOLESTEROL FOODS

The 1 + 1 – 1 Eating Plan begins by selectively adding foods that are low in cholesterol. See page 4 for an explanation of cholesterol.

Add Vegetables

Eat eight to ten servings of vegetables per day. Top vegetables for fiber and nutrients are leafy greens (dark green lettuce, collards, kale, arugula, spinach), broccoli, cabbage, Brussels sprouts, carrots, eggplant, sweet potatoes, yams, pumpkin, squash, bell peppers, and asparagus.

Add Fruits

Eat two servings of fruit per day. Top fruits for nutrients and fiber are berries (blueberries, blackberries, raspberries, strawberries), pomegranates, apples, pears, oranges, bananas, kiwis, prunes, papayas, and mangoes.

Add Legumes

Eat at least three servings of legumes per week. Common legumes are beans (all types), lentils, chickpeas, and peas.

FOODS THAT INCREASE GOOD CHOLESTEROL AND DECREASE INFLAMMATION

Step up your eating regime by incorporating good fats, fiber, vitamins, and minerals, all known to increase good cholesterol and help decrease inflammation.

Add Good Fats

Fish: Eat fish two to three times per week. The best types are salmon, mackerel, trout, tuna, and herring, but all other types are good because they're low in cholesterol and high in protein.

Avocados: Add avocados to salads for a great taste and to help your body better absorb key antioxidants, such as carotenoids.

Olives and cooking oil: Use only virgin olive oil, coconut oil, or organic canola oil to panfry foods.

Salad oils: Virgin and organic oils are not processed at a high temperature, so good fats are not damaged. (Damaged fats increase bad cholesterol.) Cold-pressed, virgin, or extra-virgin unprocessed oils include flax oil, extra-virgin olive oil, virgin or organic canola oil, and pumpkin seed oil. (Use only cold flax and pumpkin seed oils; heating these oils destroys their beneficial properties.)

Seeds: Use raw seeds, which better retain good fats, including pumpkin seeds, sunflower seeds, and sesame seeds. "New" seeds, such as chia seeds and hemp seeds are extremely high in omega-3s, fiber, and nutrients that combat cholesterol.

Nuts: The best nuts are walnuts, almonds, Brazil nuts, pecans, hazelnuts, and pistachios. Raw nuts are better than roasted, because they contain the highest levels of good fats. Walnuts are unique among nuts because they have omega-3 fat in addition to good polyunsaturated fat. Almonds have much more healthful fat than saturated fat, and they contain no cholesterol, lots of protein, fiber, calcium, and vitamin E.

Add Fiber

Foods high in fiber can also be favorite snacks, such as pears and apples with their skins, oranges, strawberries, and air-popped popcorn. Cooked whole-wheat spaghetti, cooked oatmeal or brown rice, and rye bread are other good sources of fiber. The champions of fiber are grains, legumes, and flaxseeds.

Grains: The top grains for fiber and nutrients include oats and oat bran, barley, bulgur wheat, rye, buckwheat, quinoa, whole wheat, and brown rice.

Legumes: The best legumes for fiber and nutrients include black beans, navy beans, pinto beans, kidney beans, lima beans, cannellini beans, split peas, lentils, chickpeas, and peas.

Flaxseed: Fresh ground flaxseed is the best way to get fiber and good fats from flaxseed.

Add Vitamins and Minerals

Vitamin B: Good sources include dark leafy greens, salmon, tuna, and asparagus.

Vitamin C: Good sources include bell peppers, thyme, parsley, broccoli, kiwi, and papaya.

Vitamin E: Good sources include almonds, sunflower seeds, spinach, avocado, wheat germ, and whole-grain rye.

Allicin: A good source of allicin is garlic.

Curcumin: A good source of curcumin is the spice turmeric, which is often used in curry.

Flavonoids: A good source of flavonoids is dark chocolate. Limit your portions to two or three squares per day, because chocolate contains saturated fat.

Lutein: Good sources are dark, leafy greens, such as kale and spinach.

Magnesium: Good sources include spinach, pumpkin seeds, sesame seeds, fish, and beans.

Potassium: Good sources include Swiss chard, lima beans, potatoes, yams, spinach, and squash.

Selenium: Good sources include oats, wheat bran, and Brazil nuts. Other sources are sunflower seeds and fish.

. . . .

Participants in a recent study reduced their total cholesterol and increased good HDL cholesterol when they took selenium supplements, according to research done by the Johns Hopkins Bloomberg School of Public Health in Baltimore. Brazil nuts are the richest source of selenium available.

. . . .

Sterols and stanols: Good sources of sterols and stanols are vegetable oils, such as sunflower oil, corn oil, and soybean oil. Sterols and stanols can also be found in vegetables and grains.

FOODS TO AVOID

The third component of the 1 + 1 – 1 Eating Plan focuses on what *not* to eat. Make a conscious choice to reduce or eliminate foods that are high in cholesterol and saturated fats, and to avoid trans fats, omega-6 fats found in processed oils, simple carbohydrates, sugars, and salt.

Subtract Foods High in Cholesterol and Saturated Fat

Conventional eggs: Avoid those that are not from free-range chickens. Choose varieties with omega-3 fats added, and limit yourself to one per day.

Deli meats: Avoid bologna, pepperoni, salami, and sausage.

Fatty cheese: Avoid cheddar, cream cheese, full-fat soft cheese, Gouda, Gruyère, mascarpone, Roquefort, and Stilton.

French fries and other deep-fried foods: Not sure if a food is deep-fried? If it's breaded, battered, or crisp on the outside like chicken wings, it is usually deep-fried. When in doubt, ask.

Full-fat milk, cream, full-fat ice cream, high-fat yogurt: Choose 2 percent fat or less.

High-fat spreads and oils: Avoid butter, palm oils, shortening, and lard.

High-fat sweet goods: Avoid croissants, pastries or Danishes, donuts, and commercially made muffins, cookies, and cakes.

Meat: Avoid fatty cuts of beef, lamb, pork, bacon, and duck, and fatty parts of chicken, including wings and thighs.

Premade dinner foods: Avoid prepared, heat-at-home foods like chicken nuggets and Chinese vegetable rolls.

Snack chips: Avoid potato chips and other types of snack chips.

Some seafood: Avoid prawns, shrimp, crab, lobster, and squid (calamari).

Subtract Trans Fats

Foods containing trans fats to avoid include:

Most margarine.

Packaged cookies and conventional crackers: Instead choose health-food varieties that list "no saturated fat or hydrogenated fat," and use virgin or organic oils processed at low heat.

Packaged goods: These include some peanut butters, salad dressings, and snack dips that have hydrogenated or partially hydrogenated oils.

Petroleum-derived oil: This includes some spray oils, coffee creamers, and specialty flavored coffee-with-cream powders.

Store-bought cakes and donuts, and commercially made muffins, cookies, and cakes.

Subtract (Reduce) Omega-6 Fats Found in Processed Oils

*Limit purchases of processed foods in boxes or cans with ingredient labels
listing palm oil, canola oil, soybean oil, vegetable oil, corn oil, safflower oil,
or cottonseed oil. Also reduce the use of oils in your own food preparation,
frying, and baking. Instead, use a healthful oil substitute (see page 25) or
use lesser amounts of either extra-virgin olive oil, organic coconut oil, clear
(not dark, toasted) sesame oil, or cold-pressed or organic canola oil.*

Subtract Simple Carbohydrates and Sugar

Seek out healthier alternatives to the following foods and beverages:

Boxed foods with sugar.

Desserts and sweets made with sugar: See page 25 and 26 for suggestions
on healthful sweeteners to substitute.

Low-calorie sugar substitutes: This includes sucralose and aspartame.

Soft drinks and fruit juices with added sugar.

White rice: Substitute with brown rice, wild rice, quinoa, or whole grains.

White wheat flour in foods: This includes breads (bagels, buns, tortillas),
boxed cereal such as toasted oats or corn flakes, and conventional semolina pasta.

*A recent study conducted among overweight adults found that drinking
fructose-sweetened beverages—three servings a day for ten weeks—led to
elevated blood triglyceride (fat) and LDL (bad) cholesterol levels. Fructose
sugar refers to high-fructose corn syrup or sugar that is highly processed
and condensed from fruit and some vegetables.*

Subtract (Reduce) Salt

Reduce salt in your cooking by using herbs and spices instead. For example, use rosemary with yams, cauliflower, or pumpkin; oregano with zucchini; ginger with Brussels sprouts or carrots; and basil with tomatoes.

HOW MUCH IS A SERVING?

Serving portions as listed in government food guides are not very large, and remembering to choose portions wisely is almost as important as the food choices you make. If the task of eating more healthful foods seems daunting, remember that you need relatively small amounts to gain big health benefits. USDA Food Guide portion sizes include 1 slice of bread or ½ cup cooked cereal, rice, or pasta when consuming grains; 1 cup of raw leafy vegetables or ½ cup cooked vegetables; 1 medium fruit or ½ cup of cooked or canned fruit; 2 to 3 ounces of cooked lean meat, poultry, or fish; 6 to 12 nuts (depending on size) or 2 tablespoons of nut butter; and 1 cup of 2 percent milk or yogurt, or 1½ ounces low-fat cheese.

HOW TO READ LABELS

The most important part of the label on any food is the ingredient list. There you'll find out exactly what and how much is in the food. Ingredients are listed from largest to smallest amounts; beware of labels that list two or three different words for sugar, salt, or fat so that, divided, they don't have to be listed as the first ingredient. The American Heart Association's website offers tips for reading nutrition facts. Pay close attention to the "% Daily Value" section, which tells you the percent of each nutrient in a single serving in terms of the daily recommended amount. Optimally, choose foods that contain 5 percent or less daily value (DV) of saturated fat, cholesterol, and sodium. For the nutrients you want to consume more of, such as fiber, read labels to select foods with a 20 percent or higher DV (based on a 2,000-calorie-per-day diet; keep in mind that depending upon your age, gender, activity level, and whether you're trying to lose, gain, or maintain your weight, you may need to adjust the calories you consume daily).

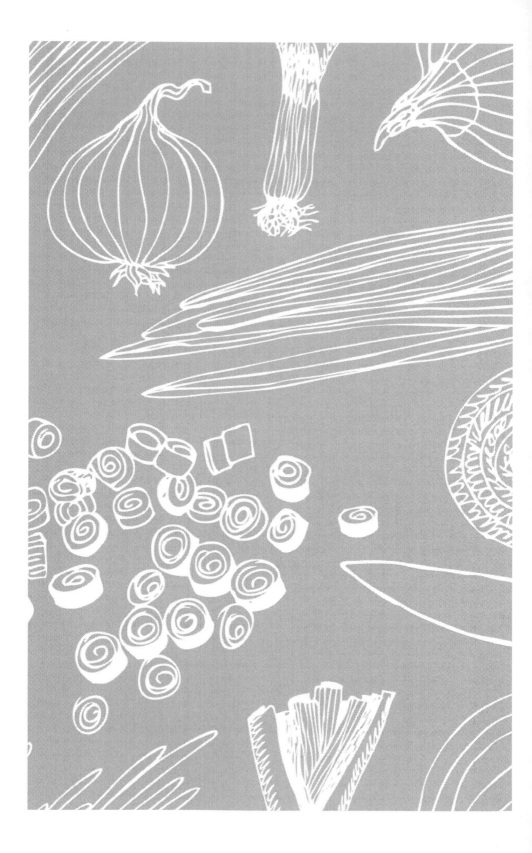

CHAPTER THREE

Making the Low-Cholesterol Diet a Lifestyle

You may be surprised to learn that simple lifestyle choices you make can affect your cholesterol numbers. Staying active, cutting down on caffeine, and maintaining a good sense of humor can all work in your favor to keep your cholesterol levels in check. In this chapter, you'll find tips for lifestyle habits that can help lower cholesterol, guidelines for smart food choices when eating out, advice if you are taking cholesterol medication, handy substitutions and alternatives for cooking and baking, cooking tips, and useful questions to ask yourself as you prepare and enjoy each meal.

When it comes to high cholesterol and heart disease, men have traditionally gotten more attention than women. However, more women than men die of heart disease. And according to the FDA, gender also affects cholesterol levels; cholesterol naturally rises as women age, and menopause may increase a woman's LDL (bad) cholesterol. Although you can't change factors like gender, age, and family history, there are key steps you can take to avoid increasing cholesterol and your risk of heart problems by adopting a healthful lifestyle; it's never too late—or too early—to start.

LIFESTYLE STEPS TO HELP LOWER CHOLESTEROL

What you do and what you eat can both be good for you. Alongside making healthful food choices, here are ten high cholesterol (and heart disease) prevention steps that will yield positive results:

1. **Don't Smoke.** Smoking is the most powerful, preventable risk factor for heart disease, and it may also put cholesterol levels off balance. Cigarette smoke lowers HDL (good) cholesterol levels, according to the FDA.

Tobacco smoke contains chemicals that damage your heart and blood vessels, making them more vulnerable to disease. The nicotine and carbon monoxide in cigarette smoke also increases heart rate and blood pressure. No matter how long you've smoked, you'll start reaping rewards as soon as you quit.

2. **Be Active.** Participating in physical activity each day for thirty to sixty minutes can reduce cholesterol levels and reduce heart disease risks by one-quarter. Exercise increases blood flow through arteries and strengthens heart contractions so that the heart pumps more blood with less effort.

3. **Consult with a Professional.** Consult with a personal trainer or doctor to determine an appropriate exercise program that sets measurable and attainable goals. Work with him or her to make small changes: use the stairs instead of elevators, walk instead of driving, and take a stroll after dinner instead of watching TV.

4. **Maintain a Healthful Weight.** Excess weight can lead to poor health conditions, including high blood pressure, higher blood fats, and high cholesterol that increase one's chances of heart disease. Even small reductions can help—reducing your weight by 10 percent can decrease blood pressure, lower your blood cholesterol level, and reduce diabetes risk.

5. **Take Supplements.** If you don't get enough fish in your diet, fish oil supplements that provide at least 1,000 mg of combined EPA and DHA are recommended to support higher (good) HDL levels. High (bad) LDL may be reduced with a niacin (vitamin B3) supplement. Also consider taking vitamin C, D, and E supplements. Inulin and other types of soluble fiber that help to lower bad cholesterol can be found in a supplement. Garlic capsules are good to take if you don't get enough in your food; multiple studies have shown reductions in total cholesterol, and particularly bad cholesterol, with garlic supplements. The herb ginkgo biloba is thought to improve blood flow throughout the body, and helps circulation by widening the arteries. Ginseng may also protect the heart and lower cholesterol.

6. **Reduce Caffeine.** Instead of coffee and caffeinated soft drinks, opt for green tea. Results published in the *American Journal of Clinical Nutrition* show that green tea's antioxidants decrease cholesterol and body fat accumulation. It is believed that polyphenols in green tea block the body's absorption of cholesterol and help it get excreted from the body.

7. **Avoid Alcohol.** A direct correlation between alcohol consumption and blood pressure has been discovered. The USDA recommends consuming no more than one alcoholic drink per day, and when you do, to make it heart-healthier red wine, which has the antioxidant resveratrol. Studies link drinking purple grape juice or moderate amounts of red wine (up to two 4-ounce servings daily for men and one 4-ounce serving daily for women) to improved heart health and reduced inflammation due partly to resveratrol.

8. **Consider the Medications You're Taking.** Many prescription drugs have unintended side effects, and some deplete the body of essential nutrients. Cholesterol-lowering statin drugs, for example, interfere with coenzyme Q10 (CoQ10) production; CoQ10 is a nutrient essential for cellular energy. As a countermeasure, you can take supplemental CoQ10 or eat foods high in CoQ10, such as fish, meat, or whole grains. Other potential adverse effects of statin drugs include muscle weakness, liver dysfunction, and possible links to memory loss and nerve damage. (See "Dietary Considerations if Taking Cholesterol Medication" on page 24.)

9. **Get to the Heart of the Matter.** Foods, exercise, and supplements can't do their job if you have uncontrolled stress or don't get enough sleep. One way to help relieve stress is to laugh. Cardiologists at the University of Maryland Medical Center in Baltimore conducted studies on the effects of laughter on coronary heart disease, showing that people who laugh regularly are less likely to develop heart trouble, or will have much milder symptoms than those who are more negative and have less of a sense of humor. They found that laughter promotes the growth of endothelium, a protective skin barrier that lines your blood vessels and prevents cholesterol buildup in arteries. Find ways to make room in your life for laughter, such as reading joke books or watching funny movies.

10. **Have Regular Checkups and Cholesterol Tests.** The American Heart Association endorses guidelines for detection of high cholesterol: All adults age twenty or older should have a fasting lipoprotein profile—which measures total cholesterol, LDL (bad) cholesterol, HDL (good) cholesterol, and triglycerides—once every two to five years. If you have risk factors, it should be done each year. Measuring LDL particle size is a new generation of cholesterol testing that can be done as part of your regular checkup. Particle size is important because people with small, dense LDL have four times the risk of developing heart disease. To determine how

your cholesterol levels affect your risk of heart disease, your doctor will also take into account risk factors such as family history, smoking, and high blood pressure.

RESTAURANT CHOICES

Food prepared and served at even the best restaurants is often made to taste good rather than healthful. Butter, cream, salt, and sugar are main ingredients in the creation of some of the gourmet meals that you can't resist. How do you dine out without throwing your eating plan out the window?

1. **Say no to (most) takeout.** It's hard to eat low-cholesterol meals when someone else is cooking. You can make pizza at home with fresh vegetables, olive oil, and a little fat-free cheese, but when you go to the pizza parlor, your meal will be full-fat and high in sodium. Consider such foods a rare treat. Set aside time on a weekend to make foods you like to eat during the week or foods you can freeze for a night when you don't have much time or energy to make a full meal.
2. **Be bold in a restaurant.** Don't be afraid to ask your server for low-cholesterol and heart-healthful menu suggestions. Chefs are often willing to prepare cooked-to-order specialties with low-cholesterol alternatives.
3. **Share.** If you have a decadent appetizer, *as a treat once in a while*, share the appetizer with your companions. If you have a craving for dessert, order a single serving and share it—divided two or four ways, it's far less costly to your diet.

DIETARY CONSIDERATIONS IF TAKING CHOLESTEROL MEDICATION

While they do effectively decrease cholesterol, taking medications may: (1) deplete your supply of nutrients, (2) increase your need for certain nutrients because they are being used more, or (3) interfere with your cells' use of certain nutrients. If you are taking the following medications, check which nutrients they deplete and compensate by adding the foods suggested to your diet.

Colesevelam: Used to treat elevated cholesterol, either by itself or with a statin drug. Taking this medicine may deplete these nutrients:

- Beta-carotene (eat orange and red vegetables and fruits such as squash, yams, carrots, and mangoes)

- Folic acid (eat dark, leafy greens, chia seeds, salmon, and whole grains)
- Iron (eat green, leafy vegetables and molasses)
- Vitamin A (eat squash, carrots, pumpkins, collard greens, and beet greens)
- Vitamin B12 (eat red meat or a take a supplement)
- Vitamin D (eat fish, mushrooms, and eggs, and be sure to get some sunshine each day)
- Vitamin E (eat almonds, sunflower seeds, avocados, and wheat germ)

Raloxifene: Used to help prevent bone loss and improve cholesterol levels. Taking this medication may deplete these nutrients:

- Magnesium (eat leafy greens, pumpkin seeds, and fish)
- Vitamin B6 (eat fish, beans, avocados, and whole grains)

Simvastatin: Used to reduce cholesterol and blood fats; within the statin family of drugs. Statin medications may deplete these nutrients:

- Beta-carotene (eat orange and red vegetables and fruits such as squash, yams, carrots, and mangoes)
- Coenzyme Q10 (eat chicken, fish, seed oils, nuts, and eggs)
- Vitamin E (eat almonds, sunflower seeds, avocados, and wheat germ)
- Vitamin K (eat green, leafy vegetables, meat, and beans)

SUBSTITUTIONS AND ALTERNATIVES FOR COOKING AND BAKING

Use these quick tips to add nutrients to all meals and to subtract what you don't need.

1. **Replace oil in baking.** In recipes, substitute applesauce, banana, shredded zucchini, or mashed, cooked squash, in addition to 2 tablespoons of heart-healthful oil—coconut oil or organic (unprocessed) canola oil—for the unhealthful oil.
2. **Replace oil in cooking.** Use extra-virgin olive oil, coconut oil, or organic canola oil in recipes for cooking and frying, and reduce the amount of oil since many recipes produce good results even when one-quarter to one-third of the oil is omitted.
3. **Replace sugar.** Use healthful sweeteners, such as dried fruits, dates, and raisins added whole to cereal, baking, and snacks to increase sweetness without adding any (or as much) sugar. Use a combination of maple syrup,

honey, molasses, or agave syrup, plus three or four dates or prunes (pulverized in a blender), for your sweetener instead of using sugar. For a good no-calorie sugar substitute, try a natural herb called stevia, available in powder form in health stores.

4. **Replace white with whole:** In baking and cooking, use whole-grain wheat, oat, spelt, rice, or other whole-grain flour rather than white (processed wheat) flour.

PREPARATION AND COOKING TIPS

Preparation is the secret to making healthful eating a part of your life. Follow these suggestions to make preparing low-cholesterol meals a snap:

1. Stock your pantry. Take a few moments each week to plan out your menus and make a grocery list. Keep on hand all spices that recipes you enjoy contain. Keep whole grains and flakes in your cupboards at all times, and try new ones, from millet and buckwheat to rye and spelt flakes. Nuts and seeds become stale and less healthful quite quickly (when fats get old), so don't buy them in large bulk. Instead, buy a good variety in smaller quantities and store them in the refrigerator to keep them fresh. Buy extra-virgin olive oil and coconut oil, and store them in a cool, dark place. If you buy sesame or flaxseed oil, keep it in the refrigerator.

2. Choose fast, simple, and healthful recipes during the week—many of the recipes in this book can be made in thirty minutes or less—and perhaps more complex and time-consuming meals on the weekend. Make meals to freeze, like stews, curries, soups, spaghetti sauce, and chili.

3. Make or buy healthful dips like chickpea hummus or tomato salsa for dipping precut raw vegetables as tasty snacks.

4. Cook beans, lentils, and chickpeas from scratch. They require soaking for a few hours (or overnight) before cooking. Soak and cook a large batch of beans or chickpeas for use during the week in soups, stews, and salads.

When cooking, always aim to reduce fats. The amount of saturated fat in meat varies greatly depending on the cut and how it's prepared. Follow these guidelines to reduce fats in meat and oils used in cooking other dishes:

1. Select lean cuts of meat with minimal visible fat, and trim any visible fat before cooking. Buy "choice" or "select" grades rather than "prime."

2. Broil, roast, or bake meat, using a rack to drain off fat instead of basting with the drippings. When you need to brown meat first for a recipe, do it under the broiler. Keep meat moist with wine, fruit juices, or a heart-healthful marinade.

3. Put boiled meat, soup stock, and gravies into the refrigerator after cooking to remove the hardened fat from the top before preparing the rest of the meal.

4. Replace meat with fish, which is good to eat when it's fatty (or lean).

5. Try meatless meals featuring vegetables or beans. Or think of meat as a condiment (used sparingly in small portions, just for flavor, rather than as a main ingredient) in casseroles, stews, stir-fries, soups, and pasta or rice dishes.

6. Grill, steam, boil, poach, or braise vegetables and fish instead of frying them in a lot of oil. If you do panfry vegetables, use just 1 to 2 teaspoons of olive oil, replacing the rest of the oil with water to help steam the vegetables when covered over low heat.

7. Add olive oil, yogurt, or 2 percent milk with herbs to whipped or scalloped potatoes instead of using cream and butter.

Bake it better. Make pancakes, cookies, and muffins from scratch instead of buying mixes that usually have added bad fats, white flour, and lots of sugar. These are three of the easiest and fastest things to bake. Remember to replace white flour with whole-grain flour, and substitute healthful alternatives for oil and sugar. Always reduce the amount of sweetener listed on conventional recipes. It's usually not noticeable, even when one-third of it is omitted.

MEALTIME GOALS

Now that you are familiar with the 1 + 1 – 1 Eating Plan, you can consciously consider each meal's ingredients as you shop for and prepare your food. Stay in touch with your dietary goals by asking yourself these questions as you approach each meal:

1. Did I *add* low-cholesterol foods such as vegetables, fruits, and legumes?

2. Did I *add* foods that lower cholesterol, with nutrients that fight inflammation such as good fats, fiber, vitamins, and minerals?

3. Did I *subtract* foods that increase cholesterol and inflammation, such as foods high in cholesterol, saturated fats, trans fats, processed oils, simple carbohydrates and sugars, and salt?

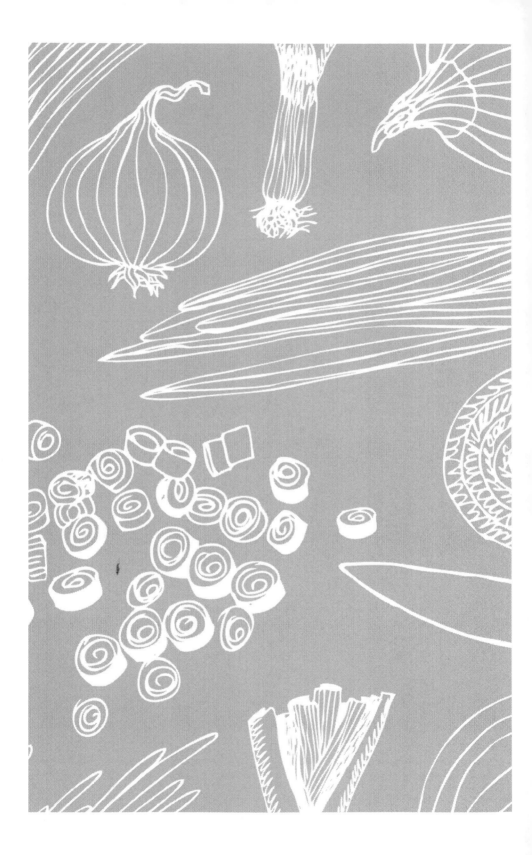

CHAPTER FOUR

Fourteen-Day Meal Plan

If you've never used a meal plan before, you are about to see how useful one can be. Each day includes three meals, two snacks (one for midmorning and one for midafternoon), and a dessert. The different dishes work together all day long, keeping you healthy and giving you lots of energy.

What follows is a fourteen-day meal plan. Don't think of this as an ironclad outline for the next two weeks. Instead, use it as a guide to help you make your own personal plan. Pick and choose among the dishes to create your ideal diet. Most of the dishes in the meal plan are recipes found in this book. The rest are simple to prepare and feature easy-to-find ingredients. Remember to consume only one serving of each meal or snack.

Welcome to your new low-cholesterol lifestyle!

DAY 1

Breakfast: Egg-white omelet with mushrooms, asparagus, and reduced-fat cheddar
Midmorning snack: Sweet and Spicy Pecans*
Lunch: Low-sodium minestrone soup with small salad
Midafternoon snack: Steamed edamame with seasoning
Dinner: Beefless Sloppy Joes* and Mashed Potatoes with Chives*
Dessert: Baked pears topped with granola and dried fruit

DAY 2

Breakfast: Blackberry Superfood Smoothie*
Midmorning snack: Apple with 1 tablespoon almond butter
Lunch: Salad of couscous, garbanzo beans, cucumber, tomato, and grilled chicken
Midafternoon snack: Popcorn with garlic salt
Dinner: Lemon-Basil Spaghetti with Salmon*
Dessert: Dark-chocolate-covered strawberries

* Indicates a recipe in this book.

DAY 3

Breakfast: Oatmeal with Pecans and Dried Cherries*
Midmorning snack: Banana and ¼ cup raw almonds
Lunch: Curried Couscous and Cranberry Salad*
Midafternoon snack: Whole-Wheat Parmesan Crisps* with Creamy White Bean Dip*
Dinner: Classic Meatloaf with Ground Chicken* and Brussels Sprouts with Apples*
Dessert: Flourless Chocolate Cake*

DAY 4

Breakfast: Mushroom and Asparagus Frittata with Smoked Salmon*
Midmorning snack: 1 cup low-fat cottage cheese with ½ cup of blueberries
Lunch: Vegetarian Lentil Chili*
Midafternoon snack: Carrots, celery, and hummus
Dinner: Acorn Squash with Tofu-Spinach Stuffing and Pita Salad*
Dessert: Strawberries with Ricotta Cream and Balsamic Vinegar Reduction*

DAY 5

Breakfast: Blueberry Buckwheat Pancakes*
Midmorning snack: 1 cup plain Greek yogurt with ½ cup sliced strawberries and a drizzle of agave syrup
Lunch: Curry Chickpea Stew*
Midafternoon snack: Salty and Sweet Popcorn Bars*
Dinner: Halibut with Sweet Potato and Lentils*
Dessert: Almond-Lemon Cookies*

DAY 6

Breakfast: Canadian Bacon and Egg Pita Pockets*
Midmorning snack: Celery stalks with 1 tablespoon peanut butter
Lunch: Farro Salad with Apples and Pecans*
Midafternoon snack: String cheese and 1 orange
Dinner: Hearty Beef and Barley Stew*
Dessert: Carrot Cake Cookies*

DAY 7

Breakfast: Whole-Wheat Carrot-Apple Muffins*
Midmorning snack: Trail mix of cashews, almonds, and dried cherries
Lunch: Chicken Soup with Root Vegetables*
Midafternoon snack: Whole-grain pretzels with 1 tablespoon peanut butter
Dinner: Linguine with Goat Cheese and Zucchini*
Dessert: Grilled Plums Topped with Spiced Yogurt*

DAY 8

Breakfast: Tortillas with Egg, Salsa, and Black Bean Filling*
Midmorning snack: Maple Granola* sprinkled over plain Greek yogurt
Lunch: Kale and Apple Salad with Mustard Vinaigrette*
Midafternoon snack: Whole-wheat pita chips and hummus
Dinner: Halibut with Citrus, Tomatoes, and Olives* and Roasted Asparagus with Almond Vinaigrette*
Dessert: ½ cup slow-churned chocolate ice cream

DAY 9

Breakfast: Silver Dollar Oatmeal Pancakes with Applesauce*
Midmorning snack: Pear and ¼ cup unsalted cashews
Lunch: White Bean Chowder with Cod and Kale*
Midafternoon snack: Whole-grain tortilla chips with ¼ cup salsa and Avocado Cilantro Dip*
Dinner: Curried Butternut Squash with Couscous and Chutney*
Dessert: Homemade Fudge Pops*

DAY 10

Breakfast: Egg-White Omelet with Spinach and Feta*
Midmorning snack: 2 cups grapes with ¼ cup shelled pistachios
Lunch: Potato Pesto Salad* over a bed of mixed greens
Midafternoon snack: Baked Potato Chips with Creamy Scallion Dip*
Dinner: Tuna with Mojo Sauce* and Couscous with Squash, Zucchini, and Dried Cranberries*
Dessert: Peanut Butter Cups*

DAY 11

Breakfast: Creamy Oatmeal with Dates and Walnuts*
Midmorning snack: 1 cup low-fat cottage cheese with 1 peach, sliced
Lunch: Vegetarian Club Sandwich with White Beans and Avocado*
Midafternoon snack: Marinated Tomato and Cucumber Salad*
Dinner: Salmon Burgers with Homemade Pickles* and Guilt-Free French Fries*
Dessert: Blueberries with Lemon Cream*

DAY 12

Breakfast: Berry and Almond-Butter Sandwiches*
Midmorning snack: Latte with skim milk
Lunch: Black Bean and Avocado Salad with Jalapeño*
Midafternoon snack: Zucchini and Goat Cheese Rolls*
Dinner: Beef Stir-Fry with Mushrooms and Swiss Chard*
Dessert: Dark Chocolate Pudding*

DAY 13

Breakfast: Banana and Peanut Butter Protein Smoothie*
Midmorning snack: Chewy Fruit and Nut Bars*
Lunch: Coconut Fish Sticks with Yogurt Dipping Sauce* and side salad
Midafternoon snack: 2 cups popped popcorn sprinkled with cinnamon and brown sugar
Dinner: Eggplant Curry with Basil and Chickpeas*
Dessert: Fresh berries topped with ½ cup slow-churned ice cream

DAY 14

Breakfast: Egg-White Sandwich with Smoked Salmon*
Midmorning snack: 1 square Cinnamon Walnut Loaf*
Lunch: Arugula and Fennel Salad with Parmesan Dressing*
Midafternoon snack: Roasted Eggplant Caponata* on whole-grain crackers
Dinner: Seared Scallops with Mango Salsa* and Mashed Chipotle Sweet Potatoes*
Dessert: Strawberry Sherbet*

PART TWO

Low-Cholesterol Diet Recipes

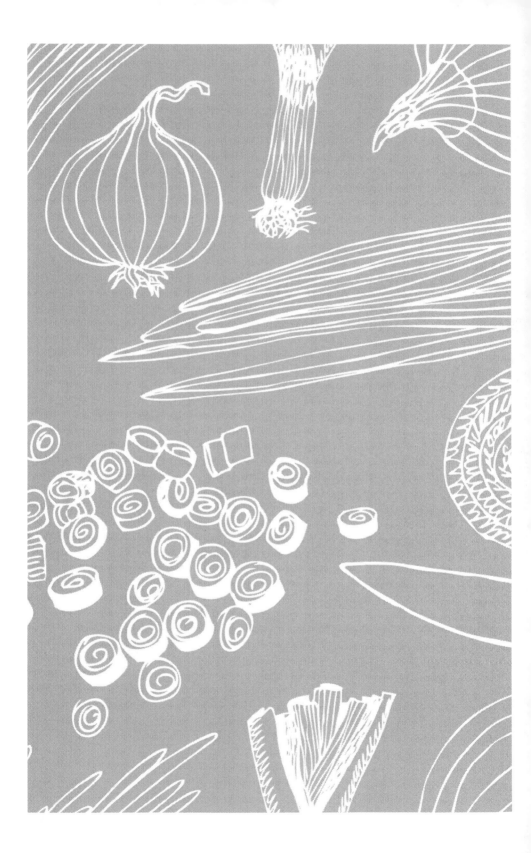

CHAPTER FIVE

Breakfasts

Blackberry Superfood Smoothie

Banana and Peanut Butter Protein Smoothie

Silver Dollar Oatmeal Pancakes with Applesauce

Blueberry Buckwheat Pancakes

Berry and Almond-Butter Sandwiches

Cinnamon Walnut Loaf

Whole-Wheat Carrot and Apple Muffins

Four-Grain Muffins with Cranberries and Raisins

Maple Granola

Chewy Fruit and Nut Bars

Oatmeal with Pecans and Dried Cherries

Creamy Oatmeal with Dates and Walnuts

Multigrain Hot Cereal with Dried Fruit

Apple Cranberry Oat Crisp

Egg-White Omelet with Spinach and Feta

Egg-White Frittata with Mushrooms and Red Pepper

Mushroom and Asparagus Frittata with Smoked Salmon

Egg-White Sandwich with Smoked Salmon

Tortillas with Eggs, Salsa, and Black Bean Filling

Canadian Bacon and Egg Pita Pockets

Blackberry Superfood Smoothie

SERVES 2

▸ CALORIES: 290, TOTAL FAT: 1 G, SATURATED FAT: 0 G, FIBER: 11 G, SODIUM: 70 MG, CHOLESTEROL: 5 MG

The spinach blends right in—masked by the banana—so you won't even realize that you're drinking your greens. This recipe calls for frozen berries, which will give the smoothie the right consistency and keep your grocery costs down, since fresh fruit tends to cost more.

1 BANANA

2 CUPS SPINACH

1 CUP FROZEN BLACKBERRIES

1 CUP NONFAT YOGURT

½ CUP FRESH ORANGE JUICE

1 TEASPOON PEELED, MINCED FRESH GINGER

1 TEASPOON HONEY OR LIGHT AGAVE NECTAR

Combine all the ingredients in a blender and purée until smooth. Divide the smoothie between two glasses and serve immediately.

Banana and Peanut Butter Protein Smoothie

SERVES 2

▸ CALORIES: 229, TOTAL FAT: 8 G, SATURATED FAT: 2 G, FIBER: 4 G, SODIUM: 113 MG, CHOLESTEROL: 3 MG

This smoothie is a wonderful breakfast-to-go when you're on the move. With peanut butter, yogurt, and flaxseed, you know you're getting plenty of protein, which also makes this a great post-workout snack.

½ CUP 2 PERCENT MILK
½ CUP NONFAT VANILLA YOGURT
2 TABLESPOONS GROUND FLAXSEED
1 TABLESPOON CREAMY PEANUT BUTTER
1 TEASPOON HONEY
¼ TEASPOON VANILLA EXTRACT
1 BANANA

Combine all the ingredients in a blender and purée until smooth. Divide the smoothie between two glasses and serve immediately.

r Dollar Oatmeal Pancakes with Applesauce

SERVES 2

▶ CALORIES: 410, TOTAL FAT: 20 G, SATURATED FAT: 2 G, FIBER: 5 G, SODIUM: 35 MG, CHOLESTEROL: 93 MG

This easy recipe packs in flavor thanks to the applesauce and maple syrup, which go right into the batter. The use of oats for white flour will fill you up and give you an early-morning fix of fiber.

1 CUP ROLLED OATS
½ CUP APPLESAUCE
1 FREE-RANGE OR OMEGA-3 EGG
2 TABLESPOONS MAPLE SYRUP
2 TABLESPOONS ORGANIC CANOLA OIL

1. Combine the oats, applesauce, egg, and maple syrup in a blender and purée until the batter is smooth.
2. In a large, heavy skillet, heat 1 tablespoon of canola oil over medium heat. Make each pancake using 2 tablespoons of batter and leave 2 inches of space between them.
3. Cook the pancakes until air bubbles cover the surface, 1 to 2 minutes. Using a spatula, flip the pancakes and cook the other side for 1 to 2 minutes, until both sides are golden brown.
4. Transfer the pancakes to a covered plate until all the pancakes are made. Serve warm.

Blueberry Buckwheat Pancakes

SERVES 6

▶ CALORIES: 132, TOTAL FAT: 3 G, SATURATED FAT: 1 G, FIBER: 3 G, SODIUM: 244 MG, CHOLESTEROL: 2 MG

Using buckwheat and whole-wheat flour adds fiber to these pancakes. Garnish these with additional berries and you won't need to add syrup.

½ CUP BUCKWHEAT FLOUR

½ CUP WHOLE-WHEAT FLOUR

1 TABLESPOON SUGAR

½ TEASPOON BAKING POWDER

¼ TEASPOON BAKING SODA

¼ TEASPOON SALT

1 FREE-RANGE OR OMEGA-3 EGG, BEATEN

1¼ CUPS BUTTERMILK

1 TABLESPOON ORGANIC CANOLA OIL, PLUS ADDITIONAL FOR SKILLET

¼ TEASPOON VANILLA EXTRACT

¾ CUP FRESH OR FROZEN BLUEBERRIES, THAWED

1. In a medium bowl, combine the buckwheat flour, whole-wheat flour, sugar, baking powder, baking soda, and salt. Create a well in the center of the ingredients and set aside.

2. In a small bowl, combine the egg, buttermilk, oil, and vanilla. Add the liquid ingredients to the dry ingredients. Stir the mixture until it is combined, but leave a few lumps.

3. Fold in blueberries.

4. Grease a heavy skillet with oil and heat it over medium heat. Make each pancake using ¼ cup of batter, spreading the batter into a 4-inch circle, and leave 2 inches of space between them.

continued ▶

Blueberry Buckwheat Pancakes *continued* ▶

5. Cook the pancakes until air bubbles cover the surface, 1 to 2 minutes. Using a spatula, flip the pancakes and cook the other side for 1 to 2 minutes, until both sides are golden brown.

6. Transfer the pancakes to a covered plate until all the pancakes are made. Serve warm.

Berry and Almond-Butter Sandwiches

SERVES 2

▸ CALORIES: 261, TOTAL FAT: 10 G, SATURATED FAT: 0 G, FIBER: 2 G, SODIUM: 288 MG, CHOLESTEROL: 0 MG

PB&J isn't just for kids and isn't just for lunch. This version bypasses store-bought jams and jellies, which may be laden with sugar. Frozen berries may be substituted for fresh ones; just make sure they are fully thawed.

¼ CUP FRESH BLACKBERRIES
¼ CUP FRESH BLUEBERRIES
1 TEASPOON HONEY
2 WHOLE-WHEAT ENGLISH MUFFINS, SPLIT AND TOASTED
2 TABLESPOONS ALMOND BUTTER
SALT

1. In a large mixing bowl, use a fork to mash the berries and honey together.
2. Spread the top half of each muffin with 1 tablespoon of almond butter and sprinkle them lightly with salt.
3. Spoon the berry mixture onto the bottom half of each muffin, dividing equally. Close up the sandwiches and enjoy.

Cinnamon Walnut Loaf

MAKES 12 SQUARES, 1 SQUARE EQUALS 1 SERVING

▸ CALORIES: 200, TOTAL FAT: 9 G, SATURATED FAT: 1 G, FIBER: 2 G, SODIUM: 220 MG, CHOLESTEROL: 35 MG

This recipe successfully replaces butter with applesauce. Not only does applesauce make this recipe healthier than its butter-using counterpart, it also helps keep the loaf moist. Serve this with a simple egg-white omelet or enjoy on its own with a skinny latte to add protein to your breakfast.

COOKING SPRAY
2 CUPS WHOLE-WHEAT FLOUR
1½ TEASPOONS GROUND CINNAMON
1 TEASPOON BAKING SODA
½ TEASPOON SALT
¾ CUP MAPLE SYRUP
¼ CUP SAFFLOWER OIL
2 FREE-RANGE OR OMEGA-3 EGGS
1 CUP UNSWEETENED APPLESAUCE
1 TEASPOON VANILLA EXTRACT
½ CUP CHOPPED WALNUTS

1. Preheat the oven to 350°F.
2. Coat a 9-inch-square cake pan with cooking spray.
3. In a medium bowl, stir together the flour, cinnamon, baking soda, and salt; set aside.
4. In a large bowl, whisk together the syrup and oil. Add the eggs and whisk until well combined.
5. Add the applesauce and vanilla and continue to whisk.
6. Gradually add the flour mixture to the wet ingredients and continue to whisk for about 3 minutes. Once it is combined, fold in the walnuts.
7. Pour the batter into the cake pan and bake for about 35 minutes, or until a toothpick inserted in the center comes out clean.
8. Remove the loaf from the oven and allow the bread to cool in the pan. Cut it into 12 squares.

Whole-Wheat Carrot and Apple Muffins

MAKES 12 MUFFINS, 1 MUFFIN EQUALS 1 SERVING

▸ CALORIES: 150, TOTAL FAT: 7 G, SATURATED FAT: 1 G, FIBER: 2 G, SODIUM: 170 MG, CHOLESTEROL: 45 MG

Just because you aren't eating Danishes and pastries in the morning doesn't mean you can't have a sweet start to your day. This recipe combines whole-wheat flour with nutrient-rich carrots to create a wholesome grab-and-go choice.

COOKING SPRAY

1¼ CUPS WHOLE-WHEAT FLOUR

¼ CUP SUGAR

1 TEASPOON BAKING POWDER

½ TEASPOON BAKING SODA

1 TEASPOON GROUND CINNAMON

¼ TEASPOON SALT

1 CUP PEELED, GRATED CARROTS

½ CUP UNSWEETENED APPLESAUCE

2 FREE-RANGE OR OMEGA-3 EGGS, LIGHTLY BEATEN

¼ CUP 2 PERCENT MILK

¼ CUP ORGANIC CANOLA OIL

1 TEASPOON VANILLA EXTRACT

1. Preheat the oven to 350°F.

2. Coat a 12-cup standard muffin tin with cooking spray.

3. In a large bowl, whisk together the flour, sugar, baking powder, baking soda, cinnamon, and salt.

4. In a separate bowl, combine the carrots, applesauce, eggs, milk, oil, and vanilla.

5. Stir half of the carrot mixture into the dry ingredients until well combined.

continued ▸

6. Add the remaining carrot mixture and stir well.

7. Divide the batter among the muffin cups and bake for about 20 minutes, or until a toothpick inserted in the center of a muffin comes out clean.

8. Cool the muffins for 5 minutes in the pan on a wire rack; serve warm or at room temperature.

Four-Grain Muffins with Cranberries and Raisins

MAKES 12 MUFFINS, 1 MUFFIN EQUALS 1 SERVING

▶ CALORIES: 204, TOTAL FAT: 6 G, SATURATED FAT: 1 G, FIBER: 3 G, SODIUM: 288 MG, CHOLESTEROL: 19 MG

These muffins may sound like they are going to be dense, but they aren't. The boiling water makes the whole grains tender, resulting in the perfectly textured crumb.

COOKING SPRAY
1 CUP WHOLE-WHEAT FLOUR
¼ CUP GRANULATED SUGAR
¼ CUP PACKED BROWN SUGAR
2 TABLESPOONS UNTOASTED WHEAT GERM
2 TABLESPOONS WHEAT BRAN
1½ TEASPOONS BAKING SODA
1 TEASPOON GROUND CINNAMON
½ TEASPOON SALT
1½ CUPS QUICK-COOKING OATS
⅓ CUP DRIED CRANBERRIES
⅓ CUP RAISINS
⅓ CUP CHOPPED PITTED DATES
1 CUP LOW-FAT BUTTERMILK
1 FREE-RANGE OR OMEGA-3 EGG, LIGHTLY BEATEN
¼ CUP ORGANIC CANOLA OIL
1 TEASPOON VANILLA EXTRACT
½ CUP BOILING WATER

1. Preheat the oven to 375°F.
2. Coat a 12-cup standard muffin tin with cooking spray.
3. In a large bowl, whisk together the flour, granulated sugar, brown sugar, wheat germ, wheat bran, baking soda, cinnamon, and salt.

continued ▶

4. Stir in the oats, cranberries, raisins, and dates. Form a well in the center.

5. In a separate bowl, combine the buttermilk, egg, oil, and vanilla. Pour the wet ingredients into the dry ingredients and combine into a smooth batter.

6. Stir in the boiling water and let sit for 15 minutes.

7. Divide batter among the muffin cups and bake for about 20 minutes or until a toothpick inserted in the center of the muffin comes out clean.

8. Remove the muffins from the pan immediately and cool them on a wire rack for about 5 minutes. Serve warm or at room temperature.

Maple Granola

SERVES 16

▸ CALORIES: 40, TOTAL FAT: 3 G, SATURATED FAT: 0 G, FIBER: 1 G, SODIUM: 10 MG, CHOLESTEROL: 0 MG

Packaged granola is often packed with sugar. Here, a small amount of maple syrup covers the entire batch. Sprinkle some maple granola over plain Greek yogurt and pair it with fresh berries for a complete morning meal.

1 TEASPOON COCONUT OIL
2 TABLESPOONS MAPLE SYRUP
½ CUP OLD-FASHIONED OATS
¼ CUP SLICED RAW ALMONDS
¼ CUP RAW SUNFLOWER SEEDS
SALT
COOKING SPRAY

1. Preheat the oven to 350°F.
2. In a small skillet over medium-low heat, melt the coconut oil with the maple syrup for about 2 minutes.
3. In a medium bowl, combine the warm oil mixture with the oats, almonds, and sunflower seeds. Season with salt.
4. Coat a baking sheet with cooking spray and spread the granola evenly over the sheet in a thin layer. Bake for about 20 minutes, stirring the granola halfway through.
5. Remove the granola from the oven and let it cool to room temperature before serving.

Chewy Fruit and Nut Bars

MAKES 8

▶ CALORIES: 210, TOTAL FAT: 13 G, SATURATED FAT: 1 G, FIBER: 4 G, SODIUM: 76 MG, CHOLESTEROL: 0 MG

It's easy to pick up a packaged breakfast bar instead of sitting down to a proper meal, but it may be brimming with fat, calories, and unpronounceable ingredients. Make your own power bars and you'll know exactly what you're eating. These bars may be stored in an airtight container for up to four days.

½ CUP DATES (ABOUT 5), HALVED AND PITTED

¼ CUP FRESH ORANGE JUICE

1 CUP WHOLE RAW ALMONDS

½ CUP DRIED APRICOTS

¼ CUP DRIED PRUNES

¼ TEASPOON SALT

¼ CUP RAW SUNFLOWER SEEDS

¼ CUP PUMPKIN SEEDS

1. Preheat the oven to 300°F.
2. Line a baking sheet with parchment paper.
3. In a small bowl, combine the dates and orange juice; set aside for 5 minutes.
4. Using a food processor, coarsely chop the almonds, apricots, and prunes.
5. Add the salt, dates, and orange juice. Pulse the processor until the mixture starts to get sticky.
6. Add the sunflower and pumpkin seeds, and continue to pulse until the ingredients are fully combined.
7. Remove the mixture from the processor and shape it into a flat rectangle, approximately ½-inch thick. Cut the rectangle into 8 pieces.
8. Place the bars on the prepared baking sheet. Bake for 16 minutes, turning the bars over with a spatula after 8 minutes. The bars are done when the nuts are toasted. Do not let the fruit burn.

Oatmeal with Pecans and Dried Cherries

SERVES 6

▶ CALORIES: 377, TOTAL FAT: 6 G, SATURATED FAT: 2 G, FIBER: 8 G, SODIUM: 280 MG, CHOLESTEROL: 1 MG

You may refrigerate any extra servings in an airtight container and enjoy them throughout the week. For the best flavor, add a splash of water or milk to the oats before you warm them up in the microwave.

3 CUPS WATER

3 CUPS 2 PERCENT MILK

2 CUPS WHOLE OATS

½ CUP DRIED CHERRIES, COARSELY CHOPPED

½ TEASPOON SALT

¼ TEASPOON GROUND CINNAMON

¼ TEASPOON VANILLA EXTRACT

5 TABLESPOONS BROWN SUGAR

2 TABLESPOONS CHOPPED PECANS, TOASTED

1. In a large saucepan, combine the water, milk, oats, dried cherries, and salt, and bring the mixture to a boil. Reduce the heat and simmer for about 20 minutes, stirring occasionally.
2. When the oats are thick, remove them from the heat and stir in the cinnamon, vanilla, and 4 tablespoons of brown sugar.
3. Top the oatmeal with pecans and the remaining 1 tablespoon of brown sugar, and serve.

Creamy Oatmeal with Dates and Walnuts

SERVES 4

▶ CALORIES: 194, TOTAL FAT: 2 G, SATURATED FAT: 0 G, FIBER: 4 G, SODIUM: 212 MG, CHOLESTEROL: 2 MG

You may not always have time to cook steel-cut oats, which take longer than instant. So on a rushed morning, opt for this recipe with rolled oats, dates, sugar, and vanilla.

2 CUPS 2 PERCENT MILK
1 CUP ROLLED OATS
½ CUP CHOPPED PITTED DATES
1 TABLESPOON DARK BROWN SUGAR
¼ TEASPOON SALT
1 CINNAMON STICK
½ TEASPOON VANILLA EXTRACT
2 TABLESPOONS CHOPPED WALNUTS
1 APPLE, THINLY SLICED

1. In a large saucepan, combine the milk, oats, dates, brown sugar, salt, and cinnamon stick, and bring to a boil over medium heat. Cook for about 4 minutes, stirring constantly.

2. When the oats are thick and creamy, remove the saucepan from the heat.

3. Remove the cinnamon stick and stir in the vanilla.

4. Divide the oatmeal among four bowls and top each with the walnuts and apple slices. Serve immediately.

Multigrain Hot Cereal with Dried Fruit

SERVES 9

▶ CALORIES: 271, TOTAL FAT: 7 G, SATURATED FAT: 3 G, FIBER: 9 G, SODIUM: 205 MG, CHOLESTEROL: 0 MG

The medley of dried fruit in this recipe makes this five-grain cereal more exciting than the average packet of the high-sugar instant stuff. At almost 9 grams of fiber per serving, it fights cholesterol from the moment you wake up in the morning.

COOKING SPRAY

⅓ CUP GROUND FLAXSEED

1¼ CUPS STEEL-CUT OATS

⅔ CUP DRIED APRICOT, COARSELY CHOPPED

⅔ CUP DRIED APPLE, COARSELY CHOPPED

⅔ CUP DRIED BANANA CHIPS

½ CUP CRACKED WHEAT

½ CUP REGULAR GRITS, UNCOOKED

½ CUP OAT BRAN

⅓ CUP WHEAT BRAN

¾ TEASPOON SALT

13½ CUPS WATER

1. In a large bowl, combine the flaxseed, oats, apricot, apple, banana chips, cracked wheat, grits, oat bran, wheat bran, and salt.

2. In a large saucepan, bring the water to a boil. Reduce the heat and add the cereal mixture. Cover the pan and simmer for about 15 minutes, stirring occasionally.

3. Uncover and cook for 2 more minutes, stirring constantly. If the cereal is still watery, continue to cook uncovered, stirring. Serve hot.

Apple Cranberry Oat Crisp

SERVES 8

▸ CALORIES: 450, TOTAL FAT: 19 G, SATURATED FAT: 1 G,
FIBER: 11 G, SODIUM: 71 MG, CHOLESTEROL: 0 MG

This crisp may taste like dessert, but thanks to the oats and flaxseed, it's actually a healthful breakfast. If cranberries are too tart, replace them with raisins. For additional protein, scoop plain Greek yogurt on top of your serving.

COOKING SPRAY
10 APPLES, SLICED
½ CUP DRIED CRANBERRIES
2 TABLESPOONS SUGAR
⅔ CUP WHOLE-WHEAT FLOUR
2 CUPS ROLLED OATS
½ CUP CHOPPED WALNUTS
2 TABLESPOONS GROUND FLAXSEED
1 TEASPOON GROUND CINNAMON
6 TABLESPOONS ORGANIC CANOLA OIL
4 TABLESPOONS MAPLE SYRUP

1. Preheat the oven to 375°F.
2. Coat a 9-by-13-inch baking dish with cooking spray.
3. Place the apples and cranberries in the baking dish in an even layer. Sprinkle the sugar on top.
4. In a medium bowl, combine the flour, oats, walnuts, flaxseed, cinnamon, oil, and maple syrup. Pour the mixture over the fruit, pressing it down into dish.
5. Lightly oil a sheet of aluminum foil and cover the baking dish, oil-side down. Bake for about 45 minutes, until the apples are tender.
6. Uncover and continue to cook the crisp for about 25 minutes, until the topping is golden brown.

Egg-White Omelet with Spinach and Feta

SERVES 1

▸ CALORIES: 69, TOTAL FAT: 2 G, SATURATED FAT: 1 G, FIBER: 1 G, SODIUM: 418 MG, CHOLESTEROL: 8 MG

Feta has so much flavor that you won't miss the egg yolks in this heart-healthful omelet. If you're still warming up to the taste of spinach, choose baby spinach, which has a milder flavor than the regular variety.

2 FREE-RANGE OR OMEGA-3 EGG WHITES
⅛ TEASPOON SALT
⅛ TEASPOON FRESHLY GROUND BLACK PEPPER
¼ TEASPOON ITALIAN SEASONING
COOKING SPRAY
¼ CUP FROZEN CHOPPED SPINACH, THAWED AND WELL DRAINED
1 TABLESPOON CRUMBLED FETA CHEESE

1. In a large bowl, beat the egg whites with the salt, pepper, and Italian seasoning.
2. Coat a nonstick skillet with cooking spray and heat over medium heat. Pour the egg white mixture into pan and cook for 3 to 4 minutes, until cooked through. Lower the heat if the eggs seem to be overcooking.
3. Top the egg whites with the spinach and cover the pan for about 1 minute, until the spinach is heated through.
4. Crumble the feta over the spinach.
5. Use a spatula to loosen the edge of the omelet all the way around and fold it in half. Remove the omelet from pan and serve immediately.

Egg-White Frittata with Mushrooms and Red Pepper

SERVES 8

▶ CALORIES: 103, TOTAL FAT: 4 G, SATURATED FAT: 2 G, FIBER: 1 G, SODIUM: 253 MG, CHOLESTEROL: 6 MG

This fluffy frittata has a little bit of everything: cheese, vegetables, fresh herbs, and protein-packed egg whites. If you have leftovers, you may also serve the dish as a light dinner entrée with a side salad.

COOKING SPRAY
1 CUP THINLY SLICED RED ONIONS
1 CUP SLICED FRESH CREMINI MUSHROOMS
1 CUP RED PEPPER STRIPS
2 TEASPOONS EXTRA-VIRGIN OLIVE OIL
¼ TEASPOON SALT
¼ TEASPOON FRESHLY GROUND BLACK PEPPER
½ CUP COARSELY CHOPPED BABY SPINACH
2 OUNCES GOAT CHEESE
24 FREE-RANGE OR OMEGA-3 EGG WHITES, BEATEN
2 TABLESPOONS FRESH OREGANO, CHOPPED

1. Preheat the oven to 400°F.
2. Coat a baking pan with cooking spray.
3. In a large bowl, combine the onions, mushrooms, red pepper strips, olive oil, salt, and pepper. Spread the vegetables evenly in the baking pan and roast for 15 to 20 minutes, until tender.
4. Remove the vegetables from the oven and reduce the temperature to 325°F.
5. In a large bowl, combine the roasted vegetables with the spinach. Spread the mixture evenly in the baking dish.
6. Break off small pieces of goat cheese with your fingers and scatter them over the vegetables.

7. Pour the egg whites over the vegetable mixture and bake for 22 to 30 minutes, until a fork inserted in the center of the frittata comes out clean.

8. Remove the frittata from the heat and let it cool for 10 minutes. Sprinkle the oregano over the frittata just before serving.

Mushroom and Asparagus Frittata with Smoked Salmon

SERVES 4

▸ CALORIES: 108, TOTAL FAT: 4 G, SATURATED FAT: 1 G, FIBER: 1 G, SODIUM: 660 MG, CHOLESTEROL: 63 MG

Smoked salmon and dill are a classic flavor combination. In this dish, sautéed asparagus enhances the pair. This recipe calls for shiitake mushrooms, but cremini mushrooms, which are easier to find, can replace them.

COOKING SPRAY

6 OUNCES SHIITAKE MUSHROOMS, STEMMED, CAPS SLICED

6 OUNCES ASPARAGUS SPEARS, CUT INTO 1-INCH PIECES

5 FREE-RANGE OR OMEGA-3 EGG WHITES

1 FREE-RANGE OR OMEGA-3 EGG

3 TABLESPOONS FAT-FREE MILK

2 TABLESPOONS CHOPPED FRESH DILL, DIVIDED

¼ TEASPOON FRESHLY GROUND BLACK PEPPER

4 OUNCES SMOKED SALMON, COARSELY CHOPPED

2 TABLESPOONS REDUCED-FAT SOUR CREAM

1. Preheat the broiler.

2. Coat a large nonstick ovenproof skillet with cooking spray and heat over medium heat. Sauté the mushrooms and asparagus for 5 minutes, stirring occasionally.

3. In a medium bowl, whisk together the egg whites, egg, milk, 1 tablespoon of the dill, and pepper. Fold in smoked salmon.

4. Stir the egg mixture into pan with the asparagus and mushrooms, making sure they are blended and spread evenly in the skillet. Cook without stirring until the eggs begin to set, about 4 minutes. The center of the eggs should still be wet.

5. Transfer the skillet to the broiler and cook until the top of the omelet is set, about 2 minutes.

6. Remove the frittata from oven. Sprinkle the remaining tablespoon of dill over it. Cut the frittata into wedges.

7. Serve each wedge with ¼ tablespoon of sour cream.

Egg-White Sandwich with Smoked Salmon

SERVES 1

▶ CALORIES: 214, TOTAL FAT: 5 G, SATURATED FAT: 1 G, FIBER: 3 G, SODIUM: 670 MG, CHOLESTEROL: 7 MG

A healthful alternative to lox and bagels, this dish will prove to be a satisfying pick for early morning. The sandwich offers 19 grams of protein, which will fuel your metabolism and give you a healthful shot of energy.

½ TEASPOON EXTRA-VIRGIN OLIVE OIL

1 TABLESPOON FINELY CHOPPED RED ONION

2 FREE-RANGE OR OMEGA-3 EGG WHITES, BEATEN

PINCH OF SALT

½ TEASPOON CAPERS, RINSED AND CHOPPED (OPTIONAL)

1 WHOLE-WHEAT ENGLISH MUFFIN, SPLIT AND TOASTED

1 OUNCE SMOKED SALMON

1 SLICE TOMATO

1. In a small nonstick skillet over medium heat, heat the olive oil. Sauté the onion, stirring, until it softens, about 1 minute.
2. Add the egg whites, salt, and capers (if using) to the pan. Stir constantly until the whites are set, about 1 minute.
3. To make the sandwich, put a layer of egg whites on the bottom half of an English muffin, then add the smoked salmon and tomato, and top with other half.

Tortillas with Eggs, Salsa, and Black Bean Filling

SERVES 2

▶ CALORIES: 215, TOTAL FAT: 8 G, SATURATED FAT: 3 G, FIBER: 5 G, SODIUM: 409 MG, CHOLESTEROL: 219 MG

Salsa is an ideal way to add flavor to a dish without adding fat. Here it's added to eggs and coupled with black beans to create a Mexican-inspired breakfast.

TWO 6-INCH CORN TORTILLAS

½ CUP CANNED BLACK BEANS, RINSED AND DRAINED

2 FREE-RANGE OR OMEGA-3 EGGS

1 TABLESPOON FAT-FREE MILK

⅛ TEASPOON FRESHLY GROUND BLACK PEPPER

SALT

COOKING SPRAY

½ CUP CHOPPED TOMATO

2 TABLESPOONS SHREDDED MONTEREY JACK CHEESE

2 TEASPOONS FRESH CILANTRO, CHOPPED

¼ CUP CHUNKY SALSA

1. In a small skillet, warm each tortilla for about 1 minute over medium-low heat. Using tongs, continue to move the tortilla around skillet and flip it over until it's soft and warmed through. Set aside and cover with a kitchen towel to keep warm.

2. In a small bowl, use a fork to mash the beans slightly; set aside.

3. In a separate small bowl, whisk together the eggs, milk, and pepper. Season with salt.

continued ▶

4. Lightly coat a medium nonstick skillet with cooking spray and heat over medium heat. Pour the egg mixture into the pan and let it cook until it starts to set around the edges. Using a spatula, loosen and lift the edges of the egg and allow the uncooked egg mixture to flow underneath. Cook until the eggs are set, about 2 minutes.

5. To fill the tortillas, spread each with mashed beans. Divide the eggs between the two tortillas. Finish with the tomato, cheese, and cilantro. Fold the tortillas in half and top with salsa. Serve immediately.

Canadian Bacon and Egg Pita Pockets

SERVES 2

▸ CALORIES: 233, TOTAL FAT: 9 G, SATURATED FAT: 4 G, FIBER: 1 G, SODIUM: 734 MG, CHOLESTEROL: 133 MG

All bacon is not created equal. This recipe calls for Canadian bacon, which is much leaner than the American variety. It also calls for one-fourth cup of shredded cheese, but this may be cut in half if you would like to pare down the calories and cholesterol even more.

1 FREE-RANGE OR OMEGA-3 EGG

2 FREE-RANGE OR OMEGA-3 EGG WHITES

1½ OUNCES CANADIAN BACON, FINELY CHOPPED

4½ TEASPOONS WATER

1 TABLESPOON CHOPPED FRESH CHIVES (OPTIONAL)

PINCH OF SALT

COOKING SPRAY

1 LARGE WHOLE-WHEAT PITA BREAD

¼ CUP SHREDDED CHEESE

1. In a small bowl, whisk together the egg, egg whites, Canadian bacon, water, chives (if using), and salt.

2. Coat a nonstick skillet with cooking spray and heat over medium heat. Pour the egg mixture into the skillet and let it cook until it starts to set around the edges. Using a spatula, loosen and lift the edges of the egg and allow the uncooked mixture to flow underneath. Cook until the eggs are set, about 2 minutes. Remove the eggs from the heat.

3. Split the pita in half crosswise. Fill each half with half of the eggs, sprinkle the cheese on top, and serve.

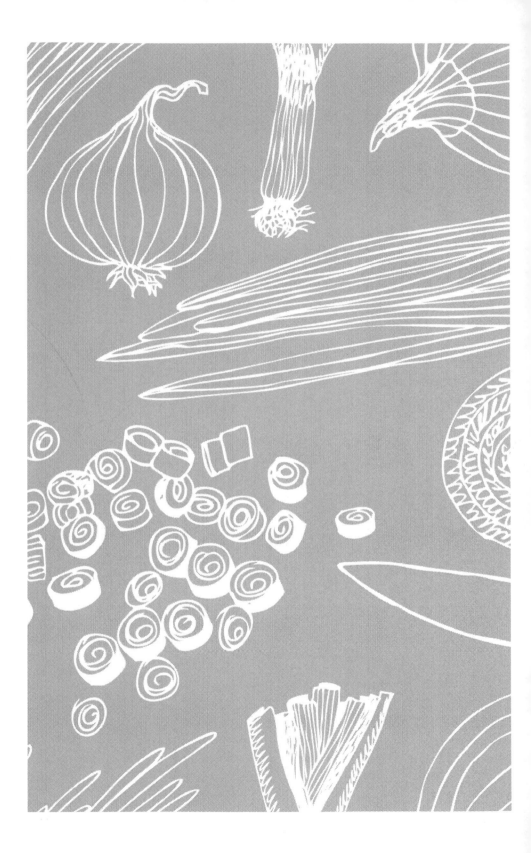

CHAPTER SIX

Appetizers and Snacks

Whole-Wheat Parmesan Crisps

Sweet and Spicy Pecans

Salty and Sweet Popcorn Bars

Roasted Eggplant Caponata

Creamy White Bean Dip

Avocado Cilantro Dip

Baked Potato Chips with Creamy Scallion Dip

Zucchini and Goat Cheese Rolls

Chickpea Sliders

Pecorino-Stuffed Garlic Mushrooms

Whole-Wheat Parmesan Crisps

SERVES 12

▸ CALORIES: 100, TOTAL FAT: 2 G, SATURATED FAT: 1 G, FIBER: 2 G, SODIUM: 221 MG, CHOLESTEROL: 3 MG

These Parmesan-spiked pita crisps are low calorie and may be paired with store-bought hummus or one of the tasty dips in this chapter for a guilt-free snack.

SIX 6-INCH WHOLE-WHEAT PITAS
COOKING SPRAY
½ CUP GRATED FRESH PARMESAN CHEESE
½ TEASPOON FRESHLY GROUND PEPPER

1. Preheat the oven to 350°F.
2. Cut each pita in half horizontally. Cut each half into 6 wedges, making 72 wedges.
3. Line two baking sheets with parchment paper coated with cooking spray.
4. Place the wedges on the baking sheets and lightly coat them with cooking spray. Sprinkle Parmesan and pepper over them. Bake the pita wedges for 11 minutes, rotating the baking sheets front to back halfway through.
5. Remove the crisps from the oven when the wedges are crisp.

Sweet and Spicy Pecans

SERVES 36

▶ CALORIES: 95, TOTAL FAT: 10 G, SATURATED FAT: 1 G, FIBER: 1 G, SODIUM: 73 MG, CHOLESTEROL: 0 MG

This protein-packed treat has hints of sugar and spice that elevate it above plain nuts. Not only are pecans high in healthful fat, but they also contain nineteen vitamins and minerals. Prep a large batch and store it in an airtight container for up to two weeks.

1 POUND PECAN HALVES
2 TABLESPOONS EXTRA-VIRGIN OLIVE OIL
1 TABLESPOON PACKED DARK BROWN SUGAR
1½ TEASPOONS SALT
1 TEASPOON CHOPPED FRESH THYME
1 TEASPOON CHOPPED FRESH ROSEMARY
½ TEASPOON FRESHLY GROUND BLACK PEPPER
1 PINCH CAYENNE PEPPER

1. Preheat the oven to 350°F.
2. Place pecans on a large baking sheet and roast them for about 12 minutes, stirring occasionally so they don't burn. Transfer the toasted pecans to a large bowl. Combine the nuts with the olive oil and set aside.
3. In a small bowl, whisk together the brown sugar, salt, thyme, rosemary, pepper, and cayenne. Add the spice mixture to the pecans and toss well. Serve warm or cool.

Salty and Sweet Popcorn Bars

SERVES 24

▶ CALORIES: 128, TOTAL FAT: 3 G, SATURATED FAT: 1 G, FIBER: 2 G, SODIUM: 26 MG, CHOLESTEROL: 0 MG

In a healthful new lifestyle, eating buttery movie popcorn will be a thing of the past. But you won't even miss it with this amped-up version of air-popped popcorn that tastes like a true treat.

½ CUP UNSWEETENED SHREDDED COCONUT
¾ CUP CHOPPED ALMONDS
COOKING SPRAY
8 CUPS PLAIN POPPED POPCORN
2 CUPS ROLLED OATS
½ CUP RAISINS
½ CUP THINLY SLICED DRIED APRICOTS
¾ CUP HONEY
¾ CUP PACKED LIGHT BROWN SUGAR
¼ TEASPOON SALT

1. Preheat the oven to 350°F.
2. In an ungreased baking pan, lightly toast the coconut for 5 minutes, stirring a few times to keep it from burning. Place the coconut in bowl to cool; set aside.
3. In the same baking pan, toast the almonds for 5 to 7 minutes, until golden brown and fragrant, stirring a few times to keep them from burning. Add the almonds to the coconut and let cool.
4. Lightly coat a 9-by-13-inch baking dish with cooking spray. In a large bowl, combine the coconut mixture with the popcorn, oats, raisins, and apricots. Set aside.
5. In a small pan over low heat, heat the honey, brown sugar, and salt. Stir constantly until the sugar dissolves, about 5 minutes.
6. Combine the honey mixture with the popcorn, stirring until well coated. Firmly press the mixture into the baking dish. Refrigerate the mixture for 30 minutes before cutting it into bars.

Roasted Eggplant Caponata

SERVES 8

▶ CALORIES: 140, TOTAL FAT: 11 G, SATURATED FAT: 1 G, FIBER: 3 G, SODIUM: 290 MG, CHOLESTEROL: 0 MG

Roasting eggplant concentrates its flavor, and the combination of capers, tomatoes, and pine nuts makes this dish hard to resist. Caponata is delicious spread on crusty whole-wheat bread or served with Whole-Wheat Parmesan Crisps (page 64).

6 CUPS EGGPLANT, CHOPPED INTO LARGE CHUNKS

4 TABLESPOONS EXTRA-VIRGIN OLIVE OIL

1 ONION, CHOPPED

4 GARLIC CLOVES, MINCED

1 CUP DICED CELERY

3 ROMA TOMATOES, CHOPPED

2 TABLESPOONS CAPERS, DRAINED

¼ CUP PINE NUTS, LIGHTLY TOASTED

1 TABLESPOON NATURAL CANE SUGAR

⅓ CUP RED WINE VINEGAR

¼ TEASPOON CRUSHED RED PEPPER (OPTIONAL)

¼ TEASPOON SALT

1. Preheat the oven to 400°F.
2. Line a cookie sheet with parchment paper.
3. In a large bowl, toss the eggplant chunks with 2 tablespoons of olive oil. Arrange the eggplant in a single layer on the cookie sheet. Bake for 25 minutes, until the eggplant is soft.
4. In a nonstick skillet, heat the remaining 2 tablespoons of olive oil over medium heat. Sauté the onion, garlic, and celery, stirring occasionally, for 5 minutes.
5. Stir in the eggplant and tomatoes, and cook for 3 more minutes.
6. Stir in the capers, pine nuts, sugar, vinegar, red pepper (if using), and salt. Cook until the tomatoes are soft, about 10 minutes.
7. Refrigerate for at least 4 hours before serving.

Creamy White Bean Dip

SERVES 7

▶ CALORIES: 83, TOTAL FAT: 2 G, SATURATED FAT: 0 G, FIBER: 3 G,
SODIUM: 360 MG, CHOLESTEROL: 2 MG

This fiber-rich dish offers an alternative to classic hummus. Cottage cheese gives the dip a creamy texture, which gives it a deceptively rich taste. Since cannellini beans rank low on the glycemic index, the body metabolizes them slowly and keeps you feeling full longer.

⅔ CUP LOW-FAT COTTAGE CHEESE
1 TABLESPOON APPLE CIDER VINEGAR
½ TEASPOON DRIED THYME
ONE 15.5-OUNCE CAN CANNELLINI BEANS, RINSED AND DRAINED
¼ TEASPOON SALT
¼ TEASPOON FRESHLY GROUND BLACK PEPPER
2 TEASPOONS EXTRA-VIRGIN OLIVE OIL
PINCH OF PAPRIKA
CHOPPED CHIVES (OPTIONAL)

1. In a food processor, purée the cottage cheese, vinegar, thyme, beans, salt, and pepper until smooth. Chill for 1 hour.
2. To serve, drizzle olive oil over the dip and garnish with paprika and chives (if using).

Avocado Cilantro Dip

SERVES 8

▶ CALORIES: 143, TOTAL FAT: 13 G, SATURATED FAT: 2 G, FIBER: 3 G, SODIUM: 244 MG, CHOLESTEROL: 5 MG

This delicious dip is a creamier version of guacamole with the same heart-healthful benefits. Make a big batch for a crowd—the dip may be scooped up with a medley of raw veggies, such as carrots, celery, and jicama.

4 AVOCADOS, PEELED, PITTED, AND HALVED
1 CUP FRESH CILANTRO
½ CUP SOUR CREAM
¼ CUP FRESH LIME JUICE
1 JALAPEÑO, SEEDED AND CHOPPED
1 TEASPOON SALT
¼ TEASPOON FRESHLY GROUND BLACK PEPPER

Add the avocado, cilantro, sour cream, lime juice, jalapeño, salt, and pepper to a food processor or blender. Pulse until smooth.

Baked Potato Chips with Creamy Scallion Dip

SERVES 6

▸ CALORIES: 290, TOTAL FAT: 14 G, SATURATED FAT: 2 G, FIBER: 3 G, SODIUM: 390 MG, CHOLESTEROL: 4 MG

They may taste like a cheat food, but there is no shame in digging into this version of baked potato chips and savory dip. The nonfat Greek yogurt gives this dip its luscious taste.

For the potato chips:

3 LARGE RUSSET POTATOES (ABOUT 2¼ POUNDS), CUT INTO ⅛-INCH-THICK ROUNDS

2 TABLESPOONS EXTRA-VIRGIN OLIVE OIL

2 TEASPOONS FRESHLY GROUND BLACK PEPPER

SALT

For the creamy scallion dip:

2 TEASPOONS EXTRA-VIRGIN OLIVE OIL

1 ONION, MINCED

2 SCALLIONS, THINLY SLICED, GREEN AND WHITE PARTS SEPARATED

1¼ CUPS NONFAT GREEK YOGURT

¼ CUP MAYONNAISE

¾ TEASPOON ONION POWDER

¾ TEASPOON GARLIC POWDER

½ TEASPOON SALT

¼ TEASPOON PEPPER

To make the potato chips:

1. Preheat the oven to 450°F.
2. In a large bowl, evenly coat the potato rounds with the olive oil and pepper.

3. Place the potato rounds in a single layer on two cookie sheets and bake, turning once halfway through, for 20 to 25 minutes, until the potatoes are lightly crisped and browned.

4. Remove the potatoes from the heat and season with salt. Set aside to cool.

To make the creamy scallion dip:

1. In a nonstick skillet, heat the oil over medium heat. Sauté the onions and scallion whites for 10 minutes, until softened. Remove the onions and scallions from the heat and set them aside to cool.

2. In a large mixing bowl, stir together the onions and scallions, Greek yogurt, mayonnaise, onion powder, garlic powder, salt, pepper, and scallion greens.

3. Chill for 1 hour.

4. Serve the dip with the potato chips.

Zucchini and Goat Cheese Rolls

MAKES 16 ROLLS; 4 ROLLS PER SERVING

▶ CALORIES: 80, TOTAL FAT: 6 G, SATURATED FAT: 2 G, FIBER: 2 G, SODIUM: 106 MG, CHOLESTEROL: 5 MG

Whether you're in the mood for a tasty afternoon snack or you're preparing platters for your next party, these vitamin-packed rolls are a tangy treat that will surely impress.

3 ZUCCHINI, CUT LENGTHWISE INTO ¼-INCH SLICES WITH
    OUTERMOST SLICES DISCARDED
1 TABLESPOON EXTRA-VIRGIN OLIVE OIL
⅛ TEASPOON SALT
PINCH OF FRESHLY GROUND BLACK PEPPER
1½ OUNCES GOAT CHEESE
1 TABLESPOON CHOPPED FRESH PARSLEY
½ TEASPOON FRESH LEMON JUICE
2 OUNCES PACKAGED BABY SPINACH (2 CUPS LIGHTLY PACKED)
⅓ CUP BASIL LEAVES

1. Preheat the grill or grill pan to medium heat.
2. Using a pastry brush, brush the zucchini slices on both sides with the oil. Sprinkle each side with salt and pepper.
3. Grill the zucchini for 4 minutes on each side, until tender.
4. In a small bowl, combine the goat cheese, parsley, and lemon juice.
5. To make the rolls, place ½ teaspoon of the cheese mixture at one end of a zucchini slice. Layer with a few spinach leaves and a small basil leaf. Roll up the slice and place the loose end down on a plate. Repeat until finished.

Chickpea Sliders

SERVES 6

▶ CALORIES: 154, TOTAL FAT: 8 G, SATURATED FAT: 1 G, FIBER: 3 G, SODIUM: 358 MG, CHOLESTEROL: 0 MG

Forget fried falafel—these sliders are a healthier use of fiber-rich chickpeas. Serve on whole-grain minibuns and garnish with lettuce, sliced radishes, and a smear of Avocado Cilantro Dip (page 69) to really wow your guests. If you're making them for yourself, the patties are a perfect protein to top a salad.

1 RED POTATO, HALVED

2 TABLESPOONS EXTRA-VIRGIN OLIVE OIL

1 TEASPOON MINCED GARLIC

ONE 15.5-OUNCE CAN CHICKPEAS, RINSED AND DRAINED

1 TABLESPOON CHOPPED FRESH PARSLEY

½ TEASPOON SALT

½ TEASPOON GRATED LEMON ZEST

½ TEASPOON SMOKED PAPRIKA

½ TEASPOON FRESHLY GROUND PEPPER

2 FREE-RANGE OR OMEGA-3 EGG WHITES, LIGHTLY BEATEN

1. In a medium saucepan, cover the potato with water and boil for 20 minutes, until tender.
2. Drain and chop the potato, and place it in a medium mixing bowl. Add 1 tablespoon of olive oil and the garlic. Using a potato masher, combine the ingredients until they are slightly chunky.
3. Set aside 3 tablespoons of the chickpeas in a small bowl. Add the remaining chickpeas to the potato mixture and continue to mash until the mixture is well combined.
4. Fold in remaining chickpeas, parsley, salt, lemon zest, paprika, pepper, and egg.
5. Once the mixture is well blended, divide it into 6 equal portions (about ⅓ cup each) and shape into 3-inch patties.

continued ▶

6. In a large nonstick skillet, heat the remaining tablespoon of olive oil over medium-high heat. Place half of the patties in the skillet and reduce the heat to medium. Cook for 7 minutes, turning the patties over after 4 minutes, until they are golden brown on both sides. Repeat with the remaining patties. Serve warm or cool.

Pecorino-Stuffed Garlic Mushrooms

SERVES 28

▶ CALORIES: 42, TOTAL FAT: 3 G, SATURATED FAT: 1 G, FIBER: 0 G, SODIUM: 131 MG, CHOLESTEROL: 3 MG

The combination of breadcrumbs, cheese, and the meaty taste of mushrooms make these hors d'oeuvres a satisfying two-bite treat. If you're preparing them for company, you may assemble them the night before and pop them in the oven just before guests arrive.

½ CUP ITALIAN-STYLE DRIED BREADCRUMBS
½ CUP GRATED PECORINO ROMANO CHEESE
2 GARLIC CLOVES, MINCED
2 TABLESPOONS CHOPPED FRESH FLAT-LEAF PARSLEY
1 TABLESPOON CHOPPED FRESH MINT LEAVES
4 TABLESPOONS EXTRA-VIRGIN OLIVE OIL, DIVIDED
SALT AND FRESHLY GROUND BLACK PEPPER
28 LARGE WHITE MUSHROOMS, STEMMED

1. Preheat the oven to 400°F.
2. In a medium bowl, combine the breadcrumbs, Pecorino Romano, garlic, parsley, mint, and 2 tablespoons of olive oil. Season with salt and pepper. Set aside.
3. Coat a large baking sheet with 1 tablespoon of olive oil. Spoon the breadcrumb filling into the mushroom caps and place them on the baking sheet, stuffing-side up. Repeat until all the mushrooms are filled.
4. Drizzle the remaining tablespoon of oil over the mushrooms.
5. Bake for 25 minutes, until the mushrooms are tender and the filling is golden brown; serve warm.

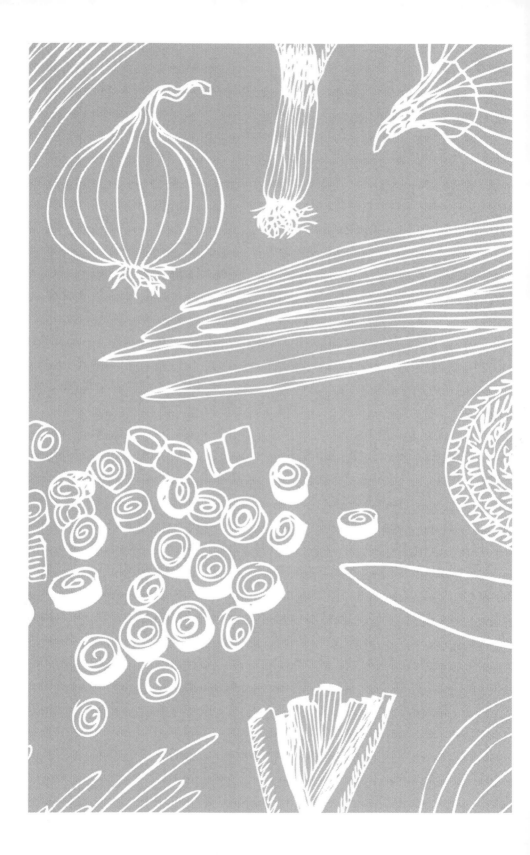

CHAPTER SEVEN

Soups, Stews, and Chilies

Chilled Gazpacho

SERVES 4

▸ CALORIES: 100, TOTAL FAT: 1 G, SATURATED FAT: 0 G, FIBER: 6 G,
SODIUM: 320 MG, CHOLESTEROL: 0 MG

*This refreshing soup is the best way to enjoy summer's juicy tomatoes. No need
to worry about precision—give all the vegetables a rough chop since they go into
the blender. You may garnish this with diced cucumbers for added crunch or half
an avocado to bulk up the dish.*

3 CUPS RIPE TOMATOES, CHOPPED
2 GARLIC CLOVES, CHOPPED
1 CUCUMBER, PEELED, SEEDED, AND CHOPPED
1 JALAPEÑO, SEEDED AND CHOPPED
1 RED BELL PEPPER, SEEDED AND CHOPPED
1 YELLOW ONION, CHOPPED
3 TABLESPOONS FRESH ORANGE JUICE
SALT AND FRESHLY GROUND BLACK PEPPER

1. In a large bowl, combine the tomatoes, garlic, cucumber, jalapeño, red bell
pepper, and onion. In a blender or food processor, purée the vegetables, working in batches, until smooth. If the gazpacho is too thick, add some water.
2. Using a sieve, strain the gazpacho into a large mixing bowl to remove any
solids. Whisk in the orange juice and season with salt and pepper. Cover and
refrigerate until well chilled.

Garden Vegetable Soup

SERVES 5

▶ CALORIES: 157, TOTAL FAT: 3 G, SATURATED FAT: 0 G, FIBER: 6 G, SODIUM: 670 MG, CHOLESTEROL: 0 MG

This chunky soup can stand alone on a menu or help fill you up faster if you have a cup before the main meal. The ingredients are available year-round, making this a soup for all seasons.

2 TABLESPOONS EXTRA-VIRGIN OLIVE OIL

1 YELLOW OR ORANGE BELL PEPPER, SEEDED AND CHOPPED

1 GARLIC CLOVE, MINCED

2 CUPS WATER

ONE 14-OUNCE CAN DICED TOMATOES

1 ZUCCHINI, THINLY SLICED LENGTHWISE

⅛ TEASPOON RED PEPPER FLAKES

ONE 15-OUNCE CAN NAVY BEANS, RINSED AND DRAINED

4 TABLESPOONS CHOPPED FRESH BASIL

1 TABLESPOON BALSAMIC VINEGAR

¾ TEASPOON SALT

1. In a Dutch oven or 2-quart stockpot, heat 1 tablespoon of olive oil over medium-high heat. Sauté the bell pepper and cook, stirring occasionally, for 4 minutes.

2. Stir in the garlic and cook for 30 seconds.

3. Add the water, tomatoes, zucchini, and red pepper flakes. Bring to a boil over high heat. Reduce the heat, cover, and simmer for 20 minutes.

4. Stir in the beans, basil, vinegar, salt, and the remaining 1 tablespoon of oil. Simmer for 5 minutes.

5. Remove the soup from the heat and let it sit for 10 minutes before serving.

White Bean and Spinach Soup

SERVES 6

▸ CALORIES: 78, TOTAL FAT: 2 G, SATURATED FAT: 0 G, FIBER: 3 G, SODIUM: 261 MG, CHOLESTEROL: 0 MG

Thanks to the use of dried shiitakes, this soup has a rich, almost meaty flavor that may satisfy a beef craving. Fresh spinach may be replaced with chopped frozen spinach. If using dried herbs instead of fresh, reduce the amount to one-quarter of the fresh herbs used.

2 CUPS BOILING WATER
ONE 1-OUNCE PACKAGE DRIED SHIITAKE MUSHROOMS
2 TEASPOONS EXTRA-VIRGIN OLIVE OIL
1 CUP CHOPPED ONION
2 GARLIC CLOVES, MINCED
4 CUPS CHOPPED FRESH SPINACH
1 TEASPOON CHOPPED FRESH ROSEMARY
1 TEASPOON CHOPPED FRESH THYME
¼ TEASPOON BLACK PEPPER
1 (16-OUNCE) CAN CANNELLINI BEANS
1 (14-OUNCE) CAN LOW-SODIUM VEGETABLE BROTH
CRUSHED RED PEPPER, FOR GARNISH (OPTIONAL)

1. In a small bowl, pour the boiling water over the dried mushrooms; cover and let sit for 15 minutes. Strain the mushrooms through in a fine-mesh strainer, reserving the soaking liquid. Set the mushrooms and liquid aside.
2. In a large nonstick saucepan, heat the oil over medium-high heat. Sauté the onion, garlic, and mushrooms for 5 minutes, until the vegetables are tender.
3. Add the reserved soaking liquid, spinach, rosemary, thyme, pepper, beans, and broth; bring to a boil. Reduce the heat and simmer, covered, for 10 minutes.
4. Serve garnished with red pepper (if using).

Carrot, Ginger, and Apple Soup

SERVES 6

▶ CALORIES: 171, TOTAL FAT: 6 G, SATURATED FAT: 2 G, FIBER: 4 G, SODIUM: 445 MG, CHOLESTEROL: 0 MG

This vibrantly colored soup may seem delicate on the palate, but what benefits! Carrots, apples, and butternut squash have a healthful dose of vitamins A, B6, C, and K, while ginger is an anti-inflammatory and aids digestion.

2 TEASPOONS EXTRA-VIRGIN OLIVE OIL
1 ONION, CHOPPED
4 CARROTS, PEELED AND CHOPPED
1 GARLIC CLOVE, MINCED
3 TABLESPOONS PEELED, DICED FRESH GINGER
1 CUP PEELED, SEEDED, AND CUBED BUTTERNUT SQUASH
1 APPLE, PEELED AND DICED
4½ CUPS LOW-SODIUM VEGETABLE BROTH
1½ TEASPOONS SALT
ONE 12-OUNCE CAN LIGHT COCONUT MILK
1 PEAR, PEELED AND DICED (OPTIONAL)
2 TEASPOONS MINCED CHIVES (OPTIONAL)

1. In a 2-quart stockpot, heat the olive oil over medium heat. Sauté the onion and carrots until they are softened, about 5 minutes.
2. Stir in the garlic, ginger, butternut squash, and apple, and sauté for 5 minutes.
3. Pour in the broth and add the salt; reduce the heat to medium-low. Cover the soup and simmer for 45 minutes.
4. In a blender or a food processor, purée the soup to a smooth consistency.
5. Add the coconut milk.
6. Divide the soup among six bowls and garnish with pears and chives (if using).

Spicy Tomato and Roasted Red Pepper Soup

SERVES 10

▸ CALORIES: 72, TOTAL FAT: 4 G, SATURATED FAT: 2 G, FIBER: 2 G, SODIUM: 127 MG, CHOLESTEROL: 0 MG

This recipe shines, especially if you buy the San Marzano variety of canned tomatoes. They cost a few dollars more than regular canned tomatoes, but they are preserved at their ripest, so the extra flavor may be worth the price. Feel free to turn up the heat in this recipe by adding cayenne pepper.

3 RED BELL PEPPERS (ABOUT 1½ POUNDS), SEEDED AND HALVED

3 TABLESPOONS EXTRA-VIRGIN OLIVE OIL

1 ONION, CHOPPED

2 GARLIC CLOVES, MINCED

ONE 28-OUNCE CAN OF WHOLE PLUM TOMATOES

1 TABLESPOON PAPRIKA

¼ TEASPOON CAYENNE PEPPER

3 CUPS LOW-SODIUM VEGETABLE BROTH

2 TEASPOONS FRESH LEMON JUICE

SALT AND FRESHLY GROUND BLACK PEPPER

PLAIN YOGURT (OPTIONAL)

CHOPPED PARSLEY (OPTIONAL)

1. Preheat the broiler.
2. In a baking pan, place the red pepper halves skin-side up and broil for 10 minutes, or until the skins turn black and are blistered.
3. Remove the peppers from heat and let them sit for 15 minutes. Peel the peppers, discard the skins, and set the peppers aside in a bowl. Reserve any juices.
4. In a 4-quart saucepan, heat the olive oil and sauté the onion over medium heat for 5 minutes, stirring often.
5. Stir in the garlic and cook for 1 minute, making sure the garlic doesn't burn.

6. Pour in the peppers and tomatoes, along with their reserved juices. Stir in the paprika and cayenne pepper. Reduce the heat and let the soup simmer for 3 minutes, stirring occasionally.

7. Pour the soup into a food processor or a blender, and purée until smooth.

8. Return the soup to the saucepan. Place the saucepan over medium heat and stir in the vegetable broth and lemon juice. Season with salt and pepper and heat through.

9. Serve garnished with a dollop of plain yogurt and chopped parsley (if using).

Butternut Squash Soup

SERVES 6

▸ CALORIES: 140, TOTAL FAT: 6 G, SATURATED FAT: 1 G, FIBER: 5 G, SODIUM: 280 MG, CHOLESTEROL: 0 MG

This recipe has the magic to make you feel like you're eating a cream-based soup, without the extra calories and fat. This classic take on a comforting dish saves time without sacrificing flavor. The squash is prepped on the stove top with the other vegetables, not roasted beforehand.

2 TABLESPOONS EXTRA-VIRGIN OLIVE OIL
1 CARROT, PEELED AND DICED
1 CELERY STALK, DICED
1 ONION, DICED
4 CUPS PEELED, SEEDED, AND CUBED BUTTERNUT SQUASH
½ TEASPOON CHOPPED FRESH THYME
4 CUPS LOW-SODIUM CHICKEN BROTH
½ TEASPOON SALT
½ TEASPOON FRESHLY GROUND PEPPER

1. In a Dutch oven or 2-quart stockpot, heat the olive oil over medium-high heat. Sauté the carrot, celery, and onion for about 4 minutes, until the vegetables are softened.
2. Add the butternut squash, thyme, broth, salt, and pepper. Bring the soup to a boil over high heat. Reduce the heat, cover, and simmer for 30 minutes, until the squash is tender.
3. Using a blender or a food processor, purée the soup until smooth.
4. Divide the soup into six bowls and serve hot.

Creamy Cauliflower and Red Pepper Soup

SERVES 6

▸ CALORIES: 191, TOTAL FAT: 14 G, SATURATED FAT: 2 G, FIBER: 5 G, SODIUM: 594 MG, CHOLESTEROL: 0 MG

With its mild flavor, cauliflower may sometimes be overshadowed by broccoli, but it is just as beneficial in a daily diet; it is a solid source of dietary fiber and vitamins C and K, much like its green relative.

6 RED BELL PEPPERS, SEEDED AND HALVED LENGTHWISE
1 TABLESPOON EXTRA-VIRGIN OLIVE OIL
4 SHALLOTS, PEELED AND CHOPPED
½ TEASPOON SALT
¼ TEASPOON CAYENNE PEPPER
1 QUART LOW-SODIUM CHICKEN BROTH
1 HEAD CAULIFLOWER, CUT INTO FLORETS
1 TEASPOON SUGAR
FRESHLY GROUND BLACK PEPPER
CHOPPED FRESH CHIVES (OPTIONAL)
LEMON WEDGES (OPTIONAL)

1. Preheat the broiler.
2. In a baking pan, place the red pepper skin-side up and broil for 10 minutes, or until the skins are black and blistered.
3. Remove the peppers from the heat and let them sit for 15 minutes. Peel the peppers, discard the skins, and set the peppers aside in a bowl. Reserve any juices.
4. In a Dutch oven or 2-quart stockpot, heat the olive oil over medium-high heat. Stir in the shallots, salt, and cayenne pepper, and cook for about 3 minutes, until the shallots have softened and are translucent.

continued ▸

5. Stir in the broth and cauliflower. Bring the soup to a boil over high heat; then lower it to a simmer. Cover and cook for 20 minutes.

6. Add the peppers with their juices and continue to cook, covered, for 10 minutes, until the cauliflower is tender.

7. Using a blender or a food processor, purée the soup in batches.

8. Stir in the sugar and season with pepper.

9. Divide the soup among six bowls; garnish with chives and lemon (if using), and serve hot or cold.

Spiced Black Bean Soup

SERVES 4

▶ CALORIES: 343, TOTAL FAT: 12 G, SATURATED FAT: 2 G, FIBER: 8 G,
SODIUM: 844 MG, CHOLESTEROL: 11 MG

*Black beans are a fiber-rich food that will trick your belly into feeling full
longer. If you're trying to ease into a more vegetarian lifestyle to keep your
cholesterol in check, they are also a good source of protein, containing 8 grams
in a half-cup serving.*

2 TABLESPOONS EXTRA-VIRGIN OLIVE OIL
1½ CUPS CHOPPED ONION
2 GARLIC CLOVES, MINCED
1 CUP SEEDED AND CHOPPED GREEN BELL PEPPER
1 CUP SEEDED AND CHOPPED RED BELL PEPPER
1 TABLESPOON CUMIN
1 TEASPOON CAYENNE PEPPER
4 CUPS LOW-SODIUM CHICKEN STOCK
2 CUPS WATER
TWO 15.5-OUNCE CANS BLACK BEANS, DRAINED AND RINSED
SALT AND FRESHLY GROUND BLACK PEPPER
SHREDDED CHEDDAR CHEESE (OPTIONAL)
SOUR CREAM (OPTIONAL)
CHOPPED RED ONION (OPTIONAL)

1. In a Dutch oven or a large heavy pot, heat the oil over medium heat. Sauté
the onion, garlic, and green and red peppers for about 7 minutes, until the
vegetables are tender.
2. Stir in the cumin, cayenne pepper, stock, water, and black beans. Bring to a
boil; then reduce the heat and simmer for 15 minutes.
3. In a blender or food processor, purée half of the soup and stir it back into
the pot. Season with salt and pepper.
4. To serve, garnish the soup with shredded cheese, sour cream, and red onion
(if using).

Creamy Potato Leek Soup

SERVES 8

▶ CALORIES: 127, TOTAL FAT: 2 G, SATURATED FAT: 0 G, FIBER: 2 G, SODIUM: 442 MG, CHOLESTEROL: 0 MG

A perfect soup for wintry weather, this classic dish satisfies a craving for cream without using any dairy. The puréed potatoes provide a velvety texture that may be comforting on a cold day.

1 TABLESPOON EXTRA-VIRGIN OLIVE OIL

2 LEEKS, THINLY SLICED

5 CUPS LOW-SODIUM VEGETABLE BROTH

5 CUPS PEELED AND CUBED RED OR YUKON GOLD POTATOES
   (ABOUT 2½ POUNDS)

2 CUPS THINLY SLICED ARUGULA

¼ TEASPOON SALT

¼ TEASPOON FRESHLY GROUND PEPPER

1. In a large saucepan, heat the oil over medium-high heat. Sauté the leeks for 5 minutes, until tender.

2. Stir in the broth and potatoes, and bring to a boil. Reduce the heat and simmer for 25 minutes, until the potatoes are tender.

3. Transfer the soup to a blender or use an immersion blender to purée the soup until smooth.

4. Stir in the arugula, salt, and pepper and simmer for 2 minutes. Serve hot.

Curry Chickpea Stew

SERVES 4

▸ CALORIES: 274, TOTAL FAT: 8 G, SATURATED FAT: 0 G, FIBER: 8 G, SODIUM: 612 MG, CHOLESTEROL: 0 MG

For those who resist adopting a low-cholesterol diet because they think it's a bland way to eat, work some curries into your weekly menu. This recipe, which may be served with a bowl of brown rice, calls for garam masala, an aromatic blend of spices—generally pepper, cloves, cinnamon, cumin, and cardamom— that may be found in your supermarket's spice aisle or ethnic section.

1 TABLESPOON EXTRA-VIRGIN OLIVE OIL
1 CUP FINELY CHOPPED ONION
4 CUPS CHOPPED AND SEEDED TOMATOES (ABOUT 1½ POUNDS)
1 TEASPOON SUGAR
1 TEASPOON CURRY POWDER
½ TEASPOON SALT
¼ TEASPOON GROUND TURMERIC
⅛ TEASPOON GROUND RED PEPPER
TWO 15.5-OUNCE CANS CHICKPEAS, RINSED AND DRAINED
½ TEASPOON GARAM MASALA
¼ CUP CHOPPED FRESH CILANTRO, FOR GARNISH

1. In a large saucepan, heat the olive oil over medium heat. Sauté the onion for 5 minutes, until translucent.
2. Add the tomatoes, sugar, curry powder, salt, turmeric, and red pepper. Cook, stirring occasionally, for 8 minutes.
3. When the tomatoes have thickened, add the chickpeas and garam masala, and cook for 5 minutes.
4. To serve, garnish the curry with cilantro.

Slow-Cooker Split Pea and Kale Stew

SERVES 8

▶ CALORIES: 261, TOTAL FAT: 2 G, SATURATED FAT: 0 G, FIBER: 17 G, SODIUM: 544 MG, CHOLESTEROL: 6 MG

If you don't have much time to cook healthful meals, try using a slow cooker. Most recipes call for minimal prep time and the results are tasty. For meat lovers, this savory stew uses a small portion of lean, low-sodium ham steak, which goes a long way without increasing the cholesterol count too much.

1 POUND DRIED GREEN SPLIT PEAS, RINSED

1 ONION, DICED

3 CARROTS, PEELED AND DICED

4 CELERY STALKS, DICED

5 FRESH THYME SPRIGS

ONE 4-OUNCE THICK-CUT LOW-SODIUM HAM STEAK, DICED

7 CUPS WATER

½ TEASPOON SALT

½ TEASPOON FRESHLY GROUND BLACK PEPPER

1 LARGE BUNCH KALE, STEMMED AND DERIBBED

1 TABLESPOON RED WINE VINEGAR

1. In a slow cooker, mix together the split peas, onion, carrots, celery, thyme, ham, water, salt, and pepper. Cover and cook on low for 5½ hours.

2. Remove the thyme sprigs.

3. Chop the kale in a food processor. Stir the vinegar into the soup and add the chopped kale. Serve hot.

Vegetarian Lentil Chili

SERVES 8

▸ CALORIES: 130, TOTAL FAT: 0 G, SATURATED FAT: 0 G, FIBER: 7 G, SODIUM: 180 MG, CHOLESTEROL: 0 MG

A strong source of iron, fiber, and folate, lentils are a low-cost way to make sure you're getting your daily fill of protein. This soup keeps well and gets better as the flavors meld together. Make a large batch on Sunday and pack it up for lunch for the week.

1 ONION, CHOPPED

1 RED BELL PEPPER, SEEDED AND CHOPPED

7¾ CUPS PLUS 3 TABLESPOONS LOW-SODIUM VEGETABLE BROTH

5 GARLIC CLOVES, MINCED

4 TEASPOONS SALT-FREE CHILI POWDER

ONE 16-OUNCE PACKAGE BROWN LENTILS

TWO 15-OUNCE CANS DICED TOMATOES

¼ CUP CHOPPED FRESH CILANTRO

1. Heat a Dutch oven or a large stockpot over medium-high heat. When hot, stir in the onion and red pepper. Cook for 6 minutes, stirring frequently until the vegetables begin to stick to the pot.
2. Add 3 tablespoons of broth and continue to cook until the onion softens, stirring constantly while scraping the brown bits up from pan.
3. Add the garlic and chili powder and cook for 1 minute, stirring constantly.
4. Add the lentils, tomatoes, and the remaining 7¾ cups broth; bring to a boil. Reduce the heat and simmer, partially covered, for 30 minutes, until the lentils are tender.
5. Uncover and cook the chili for 10 more minutes.
6. Remove the chili from the heat, stir in the cilantro, and serve hot.

White Bean Chowder with Cod and Kale

SERVES 4

▸ CALORIES: 270, TOTAL FAT: 3 G, SATURATED FAT: 0 G, FIBER: 10 G, SODIUM: 230 MG, CHOLESTEROL: 5 MG

Cod is a good source of heart-healthful omega-3 fatty acids and is a mild white fish that works well in soups. It soaks up flavors without overpowering the dish.

2 CUPS UNSWEETENED ALMOND MILK

1 TABLESPOON DRIED ITALIAN SEASONING

¾ POUND BABY RED POTATOES, QUARTERED

1 CUP CHOPPED ONION

1 TABLESPOON TOMATO PASTE

ONE 15-OUNCE CAN CANNELLINI BEANS, RINSED AND DRAINED

ONE 15-OUNCE CAN DICED TOMATOES

½ CUP CHOPPED CELERY

1 BUNCH OF KALE, STEMMED AND DERIBBED, LEAVES CHOPPED

½ POUND COD, CUT INTO SMALL CHUNKS

1. In a large saucepan, bring the almond milk and Italian seasoning to a boil.
2. Stir in the potatoes and onion, and reduce the heat to medium-low. Cover and simmer for 25 minutes, until the potatoes are tender.
3. Transfer the mixture to a blender or use an immersion blender to purée the soup.
4. Stir in the tomato paste, beans, diced tomatoes, and celery. Simmer covered for 10 minutes.
5. Add the kale and cod, and simmer for 5 minutes, until the kale is tender and the fish is cooked through.
6. Divide the chowder into four bowls and serve hot.

Chicken Soup with Root Vegetables

SERVES 6

▸ CALORIES: 325, TOTAL FAT: 12 G, SATURATED FAT: 3 G, FIBER: 4 G, SODIUM: 486 MG, CHOLESTEROL: 89 MG

Fresh ginger livens up this classic soup, which is quick to prep. Using rotisserie chicken, as the recipe calls for, is a handy shortcut. To lower the cholesterol count even more, use only the chicken breasts, which are the leanest part of the bird.

2 TABLESPOONS EXTRA-VIRGIN OLIVE OIL
1 RED ONION, THINLY SLICED
3 GARLIC CLOVES, MINCED
3 TABLESPOONS GRATED FRESH GINGER
TWO 32-OUNCE CANS LOW-SODIUM CHICKEN BROTH
2 PARSNIPS, PEELED AND CHOPPED
2 CARROTS, PEELED AND CHOPPED
2 CELERY STALKS, DICED
1 TURNIP, PEELED AND CHOPPED
½ TEASPOON SALT
ONE 2- TO 2½-POUND ROTISSERIE CHICKEN
½ CUP FROZEN PEAS
4 SCALLIONS, CUT INTO THIN RINGS

1. In a Dutch oven or large saucepan, heat the oil over medium heat. Sauté the onion, garlic, and ginger for 2 minutes, until fragrant.
2. Stir in the broth, parsnips, carrots, celery, turnip, and salt, and bring to a boil. Reduce the heat and simmer for 20 minutes, until the vegetables are tender.
3. While the soup is simmering, use a fork to shred the chicken meat. Discard the skin and bones. When the vegetables are tender, stir the chicken, peas, and scallions into the soup. Cook for 5 minutes, or until heated through.
4. Divide the soup into six bowls and serve hot.

Hearty Beef and Barley Stew

SERVES 8

▸ CALORIES: 349, TOTAL FAT: 9 G, SATURATED FAT: 3 G, FIBER: 6 G,
SODIUM: 482 MG, CHOLESTEROL: 55 MG

*Choosing to keep your eye on your cholesterol doesn't mean saying good-bye
to meat entirely. Using extra-lean cuts dramatically reduces the amount of fat
you consume, and slow-cooking the meat develops the flavor that you've been
depending on fat to provide.*

2 POUNDS EXTRA-LEAN BEEF STEW MEAT, TRIMMED
    OF FAT AND CUT INTO 1-INCH CUBES
FRESHLY GROUND BLACK PEPPER
⅓ CUP ALL-PURPOSE FLOUR
COOKING SPRAY
1 ONION, CHOPPED
1 TEASPOON MINCED GARLIC
1 CUP PEELED, SLICED CARROTS
2 TABLESPOONS FRESH PARSLEY
½ TEASPOON DRIED THYME, CRUSHED
5 CUPS LOW-SODIUM CHICKEN BROTH
1 CUP WATER
2 CUPS PEELED AND CUBED POTATOES
2 CUPS PEELED AND CUBED SWEET POTATOES
1 CUP COARSELY CHOPPED ROMA TOMATOES
½ POUND MUSHROOMS, SLICED
½ CUP BARLEY
1 CUP FROZEN PEAS

1. Season the meat with pepper and dredge it in the flour.
2. Spray a 6-quart Dutch oven with nonstick cooking spray and brown the
meat over medium heat for 5 minutes.
3. Add the onion and garlic, and sauté for 5 minutes.
4. Stir in the carrots, parsley, and thyme, and sauté for 4 minutes.

5. Pour in the broth and water. Scrape up the brown bits from the pan and bring the soup to a boil.

6. Reduce the heat and simmer, covered, for 45 minutes.

7. Stir in the potatoes, sweet potatoes, tomatoes, mushrooms, and barley. Bring to a boil.

8. Reduce the heat and simmer, covered, for 45 minutes, until the meat and vegetables are tender.

9. Stir in the peas and let them heat through.

10. Divide the stew into eight bowls and serve hot.

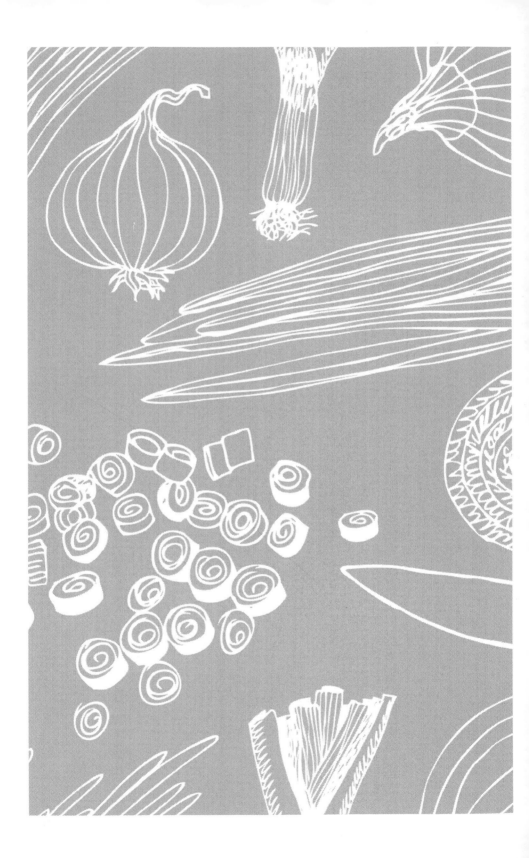

CHAPTER EIGHT

Salads

Marinated Tomato and Cucumber Salad

Avocado and Orange Salad with Cilantro-Citrus Vinaigrette

Kale and Apple Salad with Mustard Vinaigrette

Arugula and Fennel Salad with Parmesan Dressing

Curried Couscous and Cranberry Salad

Zucchini and Chickpea Salad

Quinoa Salad with Sugar Snap Peas and Mushrooms

Farro Salad with Apples and Pecans

Black Bean and Avocado Salad with Jalapeño

Potato Pesto Salad

Marinated Tomato and Cucumber Salad

SERVES 4

▸ CALORIES: 54, TOTAL FAT: 2 G, SATURATED FAT: 1 G, FIBER: 1 G,
SODIUM: 62 MG, CHOLESTEROL: 3 MG

*Paired with a bowl of soup or as part of a meal, this refreshing salad is dressed
with a subtle and sweet vinaigrette that allows the fresh veggies to shine. Using
good-quality ingredients is key to making this a flavorful dish.*

1 CUP GRAPE TOMATOES, HALVED

½ CUP CHOPPED CUCUMBER

¼ CUP SEEDED AND CHOPPED RED BELL PEPPER

¼ CUP CHOPPED RED ONION

¼ CUP CHOPPED FRESH BASIL

¼ CUP SHREDDED REDUCED-FAT FOUR-CHEESE ITALIAN BLEND

2 TABLESPOONS RICE WINE VINEGAR

1½ TEASPOONS SUGAR

½ TEASPOON EXTRA-VIRGIN OLIVE OIL

1 GARLIC CLOVE, MINCED

1. In a large bowl, combine the tomatoes, cucumber, bell pepper, onion, basil,
and cheese.
2. In a small mixing bowl, whisk together the rice wine vinegar, sugar, oil,
and garlic.
3. Add the vinaigrette to the greens, toss to combine, and serve.

Avocado and Orange Salad with Cilantro-Citrus Vinaigrette

SERVES 4

▸ CALORIES: 28, TOTAL FAT: 19 G, SATURATED FAT: 3 G, FIBER: 7 G, SODIUM: 149 MG, CHOLESTEROL: 0 MG

Creamy avocado, red onion, and oranges make this salad a party for your palate. The flavors are from Mexico and your body will benefit from the avocado's monounsaturated fat.

For the salad:
8 CUPS MIXED SALAD GREENS
1 AVOCADO, PEELED, PITTED, AND DICED
¼ CUP THINLY SLICED RED ONION
2 LARGE ORANGES, PEELED AND SEGMENTED

For the cilantro-citrus vinaigrette:
½ CUP EXTRA-VIRGIN OLIVE OIL
1 CUP PACKED CILANTRO
¼ CUP LIME JUICE
¼ CUP FRESH ORANGE JUICE
½ TEASPOON SALT
½ TEASPOON FRESHLY GROUND PEPPER
¼ TEASPOON MINCED GARLIC

To make the salad:

In a large bowl, combine the greens, avocado, onion, and orange segments. Set aside.

continued ▸

To make the cilantro-citrus vinaigrette:

1. In a blender or food processor, purée the oil, cilantro, lime juice, orange juice, salt, pepper, and garlic until the vinaigrette is smooth.
2. Toss the greens with ½ cup of vinaigrette and serve. The extra vinaigrette may be refrigerated for up to two days.

Kale and Apple Salad with Mustard Vinaigrette

SERVES 4

▸ CALORIES: 140, TOTAL FAT: 7 G, SATURATED FAT: 1 G, FIBER: 3 G, SODIUM: 135 MG, CHOLESTEROL: 0 MG

Eating kale may sound like a drag, but in reality, this super green is a true star in salads. In this recipe, it teams up with apples, walnuts, and a tangy vinaigrette. One cup of kale contains twice as much as the daily recommended value of vitamin A and more than six times the recommended value of vitamin K.

4 CUPS PACKED FINELY CHOPPED KALE

1 RED APPLE, CORED AND CHOPPED

1 CUP THINLY SLICED CELERY

½ CUP WALNUTS, TOASTED AND CHOPPED, DIVIDED

¼ CUP PLUS 2 TABLESPOONS RAISINS, DIVIDED

2 TABLESPOONS DIJON MUSTARD

2 TABLESPOONS WATER

1 TABLESPOON RED WINE VINEGAR

⅛ TEASPOON SALT

1. In a large bowl, toss together the kale, half of the apple, the celery, ¼ cup of walnuts, and ¼ cup of raisins.

2. In a blender or food processor, purée the remaining half of the apple, the remaining ¼ cup of walnuts, and the remaining 2 tablespoons of raisins with the mustard, water, vinegar, and salt. If the vinaigrette is too thick, add water to thin it.

3. Add the vinaigrette to the salad, toss to combine, and serve.

Arugula and Fennel Salad with Parmesan Dressing

SERVES 4

▶ CALORIES: 134, TOTAL FAT: 10 G, SATURATED FAT: 2 G, FIBER: 3 G, SODIUM: 155 MG, CHOLESTEROL: 6 MG

The beauty of sharp, hard cheeses is that even a small amount has intense flavor. This easy-to-make creamy dressing is low in cholesterol, and after you've tasted it, you will never want to pick up a bottled dressing again.

6 CUPS ARUGULA

1 SMALL FENNEL BULB, THINLY SLICED

4 OUNCES GREEN BEANS, CUT INTO 1-INCH PIECES

6 RADISHES, CUT INTO WEDGES

¼ CUP EXTRA-VIRGIN OLIVE OIL

¼ CUP GRATED PARMESAN CHEESE

⅛ CUP SOUR CREAM

1 TABLESPOON WHITE WINE VINEGAR

SALT AND FRESHLY GROUND BLACK PEPPER

1. In a large bowl, combine the arugula, fennel, green beans, and radishes.
2. In a small bowl, whisk together the olive oil, Parmesan cheese, sour cream, and white wine vinegar. Season with salt and pepper.
3. Divide the salad among four bowls, top each with 2 tablespoons of dressing, and serve.

Curried Couscous and Cranberry Salad

SERVES 8

▸ CALORIES: 257, TOTAL FAT: 4 G, SATURATED FAT: 1 G, FIBER: 4 G, SODIUM: 243 MG, CHOLESTEROL: 0 MG

Couscous may be bland, but the berries, curry, and citrus dressing transform it into something wonderful. Consider making the salad the day before you serve it, because it gets better when the flavors have had time to blend.

1½ CUPS UNCOOKED COUSCOUS
1 CUP DRIED CRANBERRIES
1 CUP FROZEN GREEN PEAS, THAWED
½ TEASPOON CURRY POWDER
2 CUPS BOILING WATER
¼ CUP THINLY SLICED SCALLIONS
¼ CUP FINELY CHOPPED FRESH BASIL
ONE 15.5-OUNCE CAN CHICKPEAS, RINSED AND DRAINED
⅓ CUP FRESH LEMON JUICE
1 TABLESPOON ORANGE ZEST
2 TABLESPOONS COLD WATER
1½ TABLESPOONS FRESH ORANGE JUICE
½ TEASPOON SALT
¼ TEASPOON FRESHLY GROUND BLACK PEPPER
4 GARLIC CLOVES, CRUSHED

1. In a large bowl, combine the couscous, cranberries, peas, and curry powder.
2. Pour the boiling water over the mixture and let it sit, covered, for 5 minutes. Then fluff it up with a fork and add the scallions, basil, and chickpeas.
3. In a medium mixing bowl, whisk together the lemon juice, orange zest, water, orange juice, salt, pepper, and garlic cloves.
4. Stir the dressing into the couscous until well combined. Cover and chill for 1 hour before serving.

Zucchini and Chickpea Salad

SERVES 4

▶ CALORIES: 252, TOTAL FAT: 16 G, SATURATED FAT: 3 G, FIBER: 4 G, SODIUM: 383 MG, CHOLESTEROL: 6 MG

An ideal meal on a warm day, this flavorful salad contains vitamin C–packed zucchini, which assists your body in metabolizing cholesterol. Lemon juice, Parmesan, and red onion are a perfect complement to the zucchini and chickpeas.

1 CUP CHICKPEAS

2 ZUCCHINI, DICED

½ CUP FROZEN CORN, THAWED

½ RED ONION, THINLY SLICED

5 ROMAINE LETTUCE LEAVES, CUT CROSSWISE INTO ½-INCH STRIPS

2 TABLESPOONS FRESH LEMON JUICE

¼ CUP EXTRA-VIRGIN OLIVE OIL

½ TEASPOON SALT

¼ TEASPOON FRESHLY GROUND PEPPER

1 OUNCE GRATED PARMESAN CHEESE

1. In a large bowl, combine the chickpeas, zucchini, corn, red onion, and romaine. Set aside.

2. In a small bowl, whisk together the lemon juice, olive oil, salt, and pepper.

3. Add the dressing to the salad and toss to combine. Sprinkle Parmesan cheese on top and serve.

Quinoa Salad with Sugar Snap Peas and Mushrooms

SERVES 6

▶ CALORIES: 223, TOTAL FAT: 11 G, SATURATED FAT: 2 G, FIBER: 3 G, SODIUM: 10 MG, CHOLESTEROL: 0 MG

One cup of cooked quinoa contains approximately 8 grams of protein and 5 grams of fiber, making it essential in heart-healthful diets. Fresh sugar snap peas give this dish a sweet bite as well as a boost of vitamins B6, C, and K. If you need to replace the peas with another frozen vegetable, give antioxidant-packed asparagus a try.

2 CUPS WATER

1 CUP QUINOA

⅓ CUP WHITE BALSAMIC VINEGAR OR WHITE WINE VINEGAR

¼ CUP EXTRA-VIRGIN OLIVE OIL OR FLAXSEED OIL

1 TEASPOON FRESHLY GRATED LEMON ZEST

1 TABLESPOON LEMON JUICE

1 TABLESPOON MAPLE SYRUP

2 CUPS SUGAR SNAP PEAS, TRIMMED AND CUT INTO THIRDS

1½ CUPS BUTTON MUSHROOMS, QUARTERED

⅓ CUP THINLY SLICED RED ONION

1 TABLESPOON CHOPPED FRESH DILL

1. In a medium saucepan, pour the water over the quinoa and bring to a boil. Cover, reduce the heat, and simmer for 15 minutes. Fluff with a fork and set aside to cool.

2. In a small bowl, whisk together the vinegar, oil, lemon zest, lemon juice, and maple syrup.

3. Add the dressing to the quinoa. Set aside.

4. In a medium bowl, stir together the sugar snap peas, mushrooms, onion, and dill.

5. Fold the vegetable mixture into the quinoa and serve.

Farro Salad with Apples and Pecans

SERVES 8

▸ CALORIES: 260, TOTAL FAT: 16 G, SATURATED FAT: 2 G, FIBER: 5 G, SODIUM: 0 MG, CHOLESTEROL: 0 MG

Italians have been using farro, a savory whole grain, for centuries, and after tasting this sweet and hearty salad, you'll understand why. Not only is the nutty grain tasty, 1 cup of dry farro has approximately 12 grams of dietary fiber, which reduces the absorption of cholesterol into your bloodstream.

1½ CUPS FARRO

PINCH OF SALT

4 TABLESPOONS EXTRA-VIRGIN OLIVE OIL

½ RED ONION, CHOPPED

1 GALA OR GRANNY SMITH APPLE, CORED AND CHOPPED

1 TABLESPOON CHOPPED THYME

3 TABLESPOONS APPLE CIDER VINEGAR

¾ CUP CHOPPED TOASTED PECANS

FRESHLY GROUND BLACK PEPPER

1. In a small bowl, soak the farro in cold water for 20 minutes. Using a sieve, drain the grain and set aside.
2. Bring a large pot of water to a boil. Add the farro and salt, and simmer, uncovered, for 30 minutes, until the farro is tender.
3. Using a sieve, drain the farro and rinse it under cold water, making sure it is well drained before transferring it to a bowl. Cover and refrigerate.
4. In a large nonstick skillet, heat 2 tablespoons of oil over medium heat. Sauté the onion for 5 minutes, until softened.
5. Stir in the chopped apples and cook for 2 to 3 minutes, until the apples are slightly softened.
6. Fold the apple mixture into the farro.
7. Gently mix in the thyme, vinegar, the remaining 2 tablespoons of oil, and pecans. Season with pepper. Serve immediately.

Black Bean and Avocado Salad with Jalapeño

SERVES 4

▶ CALORIES: 199, TOTAL FAT: 14 G, SATURATED FAT: 2 G, FIBER: 8 G, SODIUM: 407 MG, CHOLESTEROL: 0 MG

This salad embraces the spirit of Mexican cuisine but avoids its caloric traps. The soluble fiber in black beans helps to lower cholesterol, while the monounsaturated fat in avocadoes helps to raise the level of HDL (good) cholesterol in your body.

ONE 15.5-OUNCE CAN OF BLACK BEANS, RINSED AND DRAINED
1 ORANGE BELL PEPPER, SEEDED AND SLICED
1 JALAPEÑO, SEEDED AND SLICED
2 TABLESPOONS EXTRA-VIRGIN OLIVE OIL
2 TABLESPOONS FRESH LIME JUICE
¾ TEASPOONS GROUND CUMIN
½ TEASPOON SALT
¼ TEASPOON FRESHLY GROUND PEPPER
1 AVOCADO, PITTED, PEELED, AND SLICED
½ CUP CILANTRO LEAVES

1. In a large bowl, combine the beans, bell pepper, jalapeño, oil, lime juice, cumin, salt, and pepper.
2. Fold in the avocado and cilantro and serve.

o Pesto Salad

▶ CALORIES: 318, TOTAL FAT: 21 G, SATURATED FAT: 3 G, FIBER: 6 G, SODIUM: 182 MG, CHOLESTEROL: 0 MG

This is not your mom's potato salad! Basil, pine nuts, and Parmesan cheese replace the calorie-laden mayo normally seen in the classic iteration of this dish. After one bite of this lightened-up version—which may be served warm or cold— you may never return to old-fashioned potato salad again.

2½ POUNDS BABY RED POTATOES, SCRUBBED
    AND HALVED
SALT
1½ POUNDS GREEN BEANS, TRIMMED AND HALVED
4 OUNCES FRESH BASIL LEAVES
½ CUP EXTRA-VIRGIN OLIVE OIL
½ CUP CHOPPED PINE NUTS
¼ CUP FINELY GRATED PARMESAN CHEESE
1 GARLIC CLOVE
FRESHLY GROUND BLACK PEPPER
8 CUPS MIXED SALAD GREENS

1. In a large saucepan, cover the potatoes with water. Add a pinch of salt and bring to a boil. Reduce the heat and simmer for 15 minutes, until the potatoes are tender.
2. Using a slotted spoon, remove the potatoes from the water.
3. Reserve the cooking water and bring it to a boil again.
4. Add the green beans and cook for 3 minutes. Drain the green beans in a colander and rinse under cold water. Set the beans aside.
5. Using a food processor, blend the basil, olive oil, pine nuts, Parmesan cheese, garlic, and a pinch of salt and pepper. Pulse until the pesto is smooth.
6. In a large mixing bowl, toss the warm potatoes and beans with the pesto. Serve on 1 cup of mixed greens.

CHAPTER NINE

Side Dishes

Roasted Carrots with Fresh Dill

Kale Sautéed with Garlic and Olive Oil

Sugar Snap Peas with Mint and Garlic

Green Beans with Almonds and Lemon

Roasted Asparagus with Almond Vinaigrette

Corn on the Cob with Spicy-Smoky Butter

Coleslaw with Apples and Walnuts

Brussels Sprouts with Apples

Bok Choy with Mushrooms

Beets with Greek Yogurt Dressing

Guilt-Free French Fries

Mashed Chipotle Sweet Potatoes

Mashed Potatoes with Chives

Creamed Spinach

Chickpeas with Raisins and Cilantro

White Beans with Rosemary and Garlic

Baked Beans 'n' Greens

Quinoa with Lemon and Fresh Herbs

Couscous with Squash, Zucchini, and Dried Cranberries

Broccolini with Leeks and Bacon

Roasted Carrots with Fresh Dill

SERVES 6

▶ CALORIES: 110, TOTAL FAT: 7 G, SATURATED FAT: 1 G, FIBER: 4 G, SODIUM: 484 MG, CHOLESTEROL: 0 MG

Fresh dill can have a strong flavor, so it works best when paired with more mellow foods, like carrots and olive oil. This dish is high in nutrients; a single carrot has more than 200 percent of your daily requirement for vitamin A, which is beneficial for many things, including vision.

12 CARROTS, PEELED
3 TABLESPOONS EXTRA-VIRGIN OLIVE OIL
1¼ TEASPOON SALT
½ TEASPOON FRESHLY GROUND BLACK PEPPER
2 TABLESPOONS MINCED FRESH DILL

1. Preheat the oven to 400°F.
2. Slice the carrots diagonally into 1½-inch pieces.
3. Toss the carrots in a medium bowl with the olive oil, salt, and pepper.
4. Place the carrots in a baking pan and spread them in an even layer.
5. Roast the carrots in the oven for 20 minutes, or until browned and tender.
6. Toss the carrots with the dill and serve.

Kale Sautéed with Garlic and Olive Oil

SERVES 4

▶ CALORIES: 178, TOTAL FAT: 11 G, SATURATED FAT: 2 G, FIBER: 4 G, SODIUM: 336 MG, CHOLESTEROL: 0 MG

Kale is easy to work with if you remember that the most important thing is to cut away the tough center rib. If you don't have vegetable stock, you may use water here.

3 TABLESPOONS EXTRA-VIRGIN OLIVE OIL

2 GARLIC CLOVES, THINLY SLICED

½ CUP LOW-SODIUM VEGETABLE STOCK

1½ POUNDS KALE, STEMMED AND DERIBBED,
    LEAVES COARSELY CHOPPED

SALT AND FRESHLY GROUND BLACK PEPPER

2 TABLESPOONS RED WINE VINEGAR

1. In a large saucepan, heat the olive oil over medium-high heat. Add the garlic and cook until soft but not yet browned, about 1 minute.

2. Raise the heat to high and add the stock and kale. Cover and cook for 5 minutes.

3. Remove the cover and continue to cook, stirring regularly, until the liquid has evaporated.

4. Season with salt and pepper, stir in the vinegar, and serve.

Sugar Snap Peas with Mint and Garlic

SERVES 6

▶ CALORIES: 94, TOTAL FAT: 3 G, SATURATED FAT: 0 G, FIBER: 5 G, SODIUM: 200 MG, CHOLESTEROL: 0 MG

Sugar snap peas are now a common vegetable in the supermarket produce aisle. This recipe combines them with regular peas for a bright green dish. If fresh peas aren't in season, frozen peas are fine, but make sure to thaw them first.

1 POUND SUGAR SNAP PEAS

1 TABLESPOON ORGANIC CANOLA OIL

2 GARLIC CLOVES, HALVED

2 CUPS FRESH PEAS

¼ CUP FRESH MINT LEAVES, CHOPPED

½ TEASPOON SUGAR

½ TEASPOON SALT

1. Fill a large saucepan with water and place it over high heat until it boils.
2. Add the sugar snap peas and cook 2 to 3 minutes. Drain and rinse the sugar snap peas under running cold water to stop cooking.
3. In a large skillet over medium-low heat, heat the oil. Add the garlic and sauté until golden, about 1 minute.
4. Remove the skillet from the heat and discard the garlic. Add the sugar snap peas and fresh peas to the oil and cook until tender, 3 to 5 minutes.
5. Remove the peas from the heat and stir in the mint, sugar, and salt. Serve immediately.

Green Beans with Almonds and Lemon

SERVES 4

▶ CALORIES: 59, TOTAL FAT: 3 G, SATURATED FAT: 1 G, FIBER: 2 G, SODIUM: 155 MG, CHOLESTEROL: 0 MG

Green beans are delicious in a casserole with cream of mushroom soup and fried onions, but this lighter version lets the natural sweetness of the beans shine. Lemon juice adds tartness and almonds add a nice crunch.

1 POUND GREEN BEANS
2 TABLESPOONS CHOPPED FRESH FLAT-LEAF PARSLEY
1 TABLESPOON SLICED ALMONDS, TOASTED
¼ TEASPOON GRATED LEMON ZEST
1½ TEASPOONS FRESH LEMON JUICE
1 TEASPOON EXTRA-VIRGIN OLIVE OIL
¼ TEASPOON SALT
⅛ TEASPOON FRESHLY GROUND BLACK PEPPER
1 GARLIC CLOVE, MINCED

1. Fill a medium pot with 2 inches of water. Place a steamer basket in the pot, making sure water is below the bottom of the basket. Bring the water to a boil and place green beans in the steamer. Cover and steam the green beans for 7 minutes or until crisp-tender.
2. In a large bowl, combine the parsley, almonds, lemon zest, lemon juice, olive oil, salt, pepper, and garlic.
3. Add the green beans, toss gently to combine, and serve.

Roasted Asparagus with Almond Vinaigrette

SERVES 4

▸ CALORIES: 110, TOTAL FAT: 5 G, SATURATED FAT: 1 G, FIBER: 6 G, SODIUM: 125 MG, CHOLESTEROL: 0 MG

Blanched almonds have been cooked in boiling water briefly so their skins may be removed. Try other garnishes here, too, like basil, mint, or parsley.

2 POUNDS ASPARAGUS, ENDS TRIMMED
1 TABLESPOON EXTRA-VIRGIN OLIVE OIL
SALT AND FRESHLY GROUND BLACK PEPPER
6 TABLESPOONS BLANCHED SLICED ALMONDS
1½ TABLESPOONS LEMON JUICE
¼ TEASPOON SUGAR
6 TABLESPOONS WATER
1½ TEASPOONS LEMON ZEST, FOR GARNISH

1. Preheat the oven to 425°F.
2. Place the asparagus on a baking sheet lined with parchment paper. Drizzle with the olive oil and season with salt and pepper. Roast until tender, about 15 minutes.
3. In a blender, combine 5 tablespoons of the almonds, the lemon juice, sugar, and water. Blend until smooth. Season with salt.
4. Pour the sauce onto a platter, and place asparagus on top. Garnish with the lemon zest and the remaining tablespoon of almonds, and serve.

Corn on the Cob with Spicy-Smoky Butter

SERVES 4

▸ CALORIES: 129, TOTAL FAT: 7 G, SATURATED FAT: 4 G, FIBER: 2 G, SODIUM: 222 MG, CHOLESTEROL: 15 MG

Fresh grilled corn is delicious by itself, but in this recipe it gets even better with the flavors of lime and chipotle chiles. You may also substitute 1/4 teaspoon ground chipotle pepper for the chipotle chile in adobo sauce.

4 EARS FRESH CORN, HUSKED
2 TABLESPOONS BUTTER, AT ROOM TEMPERATURE
¼ TEASPOON FRESHLY GRATED LIME ZEST
1 TEASPOON LIME JUICE
½ TEASPOON MINCED CHIPOTLE CHILE IN ADOBO SAUCE
¼ TEASPOON ADOBO SAUCE FROM THE CAN
½ TEASPOON SALT

1. Preheat the grill to high.
2. Wrap each ear in aluminum foil and grill for 10 minutes, turning frequently. Remove the corn from grill and leave them in the foil.
3. In a small bowl, combine the butter, lime zest, lime juice, chipotle chile, adobo sauce, and salt.
4. Unwrap the corn and serve with the butter mixture on the side.

Coleslaw with Apples and Walnuts

▶ CALORIES: 120, TOTAL FAT: 8 G, SATURATED FAT: 0 G, FIBER: 3 G, SODIUM: 70 MG, CHOLESTEROL: 0 MG

Shredded mixed cabbage may be found in bags in the supermarket produce aisle. You may also shred the heads yourself, using the shredding attachment of a food processor. Don't forget that you'll get the same result using a box grater or a large knife.

2 CUPS SHREDDED GREEN CABBAGE

2 CUPS SHREDDED RED CABBAGE

1 TABLESPOON APPLE CIDER VINEGAR

⅛ TEASPOON SALT

⅛ TEASPOON FRESHLY GROUND BLACK PEPPER

2 GALA APPLES, CORED AND VERY THINLY SLICED

½ CUP WALNUTS, TOASTED AND CHOPPED

1. In a large bowl, toss together the green cabbage, red cabbage, vinegar, salt, and pepper.
2. Add the apples and walnuts; toss and serve.

Brussels Sprouts with Apples

SERVES 4

▶ CALORIES: 80, TOTAL FAT: 0 G, SATURATED FAT: 0 G, FIBER: 4 G,
SODIUM: 140 MG, CHOLESTEROL: 0 MG

When the weather turns crisp, Brussels sprouts and apples come together in an ideal side dish for roasted meat. Use an apple that keeps its shape when cooked; Gala, Honeycrisp, or Braeburn give perfect results.

1 POUND BRUSSELS SPROUTS

2 SHALLOTS, CUT INTO ¼-INCH-THICK RINGS

2 APPLES, CORED AND CUT INTO ¼-INCH-THICK PIECES

½ CUP WATER

4 TABLESPOONS CIDER VINEGAR

¼ TEASPOON SALT

½ TEASPOON FRESHLY GROUND BLACK PEPPER

4 SPRIGS FRESH THYME LEAVES

1. Trim the Brussels sprouts and cut them into quarters.
2. Heat a large high-sided sauté pan over high heat. Add the shallots and cook, stirring constantly, for 2 minutes.
3. Add the apples and ¼ cup of water. Cook until the liquid is reduced by half, about 2 minutes, scraping up any brown bits from the bottom of the pan.
4. Add the Brussels sprouts, the remaining ¼ cup of water, 2 tablespoons of vinegar, salt, and pepper. Reduce the heat to medium, cover, and simmer until the sprouts and apples are tender, stirring occasionally, about 15 minutes.
5. Uncover and stir in the remaining 2 tablespoons of vinegar and the thyme. Scrape up any bits from the bottom of the pan and cook until the liquid is almost completely evaporated. Serve immediately.

Bok Choy with Mushrooms

SERVES 4

▶ CALORIES: 250, TOTAL FAT: 4 G, SATURATED FAT: 0 G, FIBER: 10 G, SODIUM: 210 MG, CHOLESTEROL: 0 MG

Bok choy is the most common Chinese vegetable. In this dish, use shoyu (soy sauce made from soybeans and wheat) or tamari (made with soybeans). Tahini, the peanut butter of the Middle East, is made from sesame seeds. It adds creaminess here.

1 POUND BABY BOK CHOY, HALVED LENGTHWISE

½ CUP WATER

8 OUNCES SHIITAKE MUSHROOMS, STEMMED AND SLICED

2 TABLESPOONS FRESH ORANGE JUICE

1 TABLESPOON TAHINI

1½ TEASPOONS LOW-SODIUM SHOYU OR TAMARI

½ TEASPOON GRATED FRESH GINGER

4 CARROTS, PEELED AND SHREDDED

1 TABLESPOON TOASTED SESAME SEEDS, FOR GARNISH

1. Prepare an ice bath by filling a large bowl with ice cubes and water.
2. Place 1 inch of water in a large pot and bring it to a simmer over high heat. Place the bok choy in a steamer basket and lower it into the pot over the simmering water (the water should not touch the basket). Reduce the heat to medium-low, cover, and let the bok choy steam for about 10 minutes or until it is crisp-tender.
3. Transfer the bok choy to the ice bath to stop the cooking. Drain well.
4. In a large skillet over medium-high heat, bring the ½ cup of water to a simmer. Add the mushrooms, cover, and reduce the heat to medium. Cook for 6 minutes or until the mushrooms are tender, stirring once halfway through cooking.
5. In a large bowl, whisk together the orange juice, tahini, tamari, and ginger. Add the bok choy, mushrooms, and carrots and toss to coat.
6. Garnish with the sesame seeds and serve immediately.

Beets with Greek Yogurt Dressing

SERVES 4

▶ CALORIES: 70, TOTAL FAT: 4 G, SATURATED FAT: 1 G, FIBER: 2 G, SODIUM: 162 MG, CHOLESTEROL: 1 MG

Cooking the beets and garlic in the microwave saves time. If you'd like to use a conventional oven instead, wrap each beet and garlic clove in aluminum foil and bake at 400°F for an hour. The yogurt dressing may be made in advance and refrigerated. Let the dressing come to room temperature before using.

3 GARLIC CLOVES, UNPEELED
2 BEETS (ABOUT 1 POUND)
⅓ CUP 2 PERCENT PLAIN GREEK YOGURT
1 TABLESPOON LOW-SODIUM VEGETABLE BROTH OR WATER
2 TEASPOONS WHITE BALSAMIC VINEGAR
2 TEASPOONS EXTRA-VIRGIN OLIVE OIL
SALT AND FRESHLY GROUND BLACK PEPPER
2 TABLESPOONS FRESH MINT LEAVES
1 TABLESPOON UNSALTED PISTACHIOS, CHOPPED

1. Wrap the garlic cloves in a piece of parchment paper and wrap each beet in parchment paper. Place the garlic and beets in a microwave-safe dish and cook for 3 minutes.
2. Remove the garlic and set aside, keeping it wrapped.
3. Continue to cook the beets for 2-minute intervals until they are easily pierced with a knife, 8 to 10 minutes. Let them sit in parchment paper to finish cooking for about 15 minutes, until cool enough to handle.
4. In a small bowl, whisk together the yogurt, broth, vinegar, oil, and a large pinch of salt.

continued ▶

5. Peel the garlic cloves, mash them with a fork, and whisk them into the vinaigrette. Season with salt and pepper.

6. Peel the beets and cut them into wedges.

7. Arrange the beet wedges on a platter, drizzle them with the vinaigrette, and sprinkle them with mint and pistachios. Serve warm.

Guilt-Free French Fries

SERVES 6

▸ CALORIES: 110, TOTAL FAT: 0 G, SATURATED FAT: 0 G, FIBER: 2 G, SODIUM: 15 MG, CHOLESTEROL: 0 MG

The perfect accompaniment to burgers, French fries are also high in saturated fat from being deep-fried. This version cooks the fries in a very hot oven to create crispiness without fat. If you don't want them spicy, use curry powder instead of chili powder.

2 POUNDS RUSSET POTATOES

2 TABLESPOONS LOW-SODIUM VEGETABLE BROTH

4 GARLIC CLOVES, MINCED

2 TEASPOONS ONION POWDER

½ TEASPOON CHILI POWDER

1. Preheat the oven to 400°F.

2. Line two baking sheets with parchment paper.

3. Slice the potatoes into thin matchsticks and place them in a large bowl with the broth. Toss the potatoes until coated.

4. Add the garlic, onion powder, and chili powder. Toss to distribute the seasonings.

5. Place the potatoes in a single layer on baking sheets.

6. Bake the potatoes for 15 minutes. Turn the potatoes with a spatula and continue baking for 15 to 20 minutes or until crisp and golden. Serve hot.

Mashed Chipotle Sweet Potatoes

SERVES 4

▶ CALORIES: 152, TOTAL FAT: 7 G, SATURATED FAT: 4 G, FIBER: 4 G, SODIUM: 335 MG, CHOLESTEROL: 15 MG

This recipe uses canned chipotle peppers in adobo sauce, which may be found in the Mexican food section of most supermarkets. You'll need only one of the peppers and some sauce for this recipe, but the rest may be frozen for later use.

2 SWEET POTATOES, PEELED AND CUBED
2 TABLESPOONS UNSALTED BUTTER
1 WHOLE CHIPOTLE PEPPER IN ADOBO SAUCE, CHOPPED
1 TEASPOON ADOBO SAUCE FROM THE CAN
½ TEASPOON SALT

1. Place 1 inch of water in a large pot and bring it to a simmer. Place the cubed potatoes in a steamer basket and lower it into the pot over the simmering water (do not let the water touch the steamer basket). Cover and steam for 20 minutes or until the potatoes are tender.
2. Place the potatoes in a medium bowl, add the butter, and mash.
3. Add the chipotle pepper, adobo sauce, and salt, and stir to combine. Serve immediately.

Mashed Potatoes with Chives

SERVES 10

▸ CALORIES: 172, TOTAL FAT: 3 G, SATURATED FAT: 2 G, FIBER: 3 G, SODIUM: 399 MG, CHOLESTEROL: 9 MG

Mashed potatoes go well with almost everything, from roast turkey to meatloaf. This version gets its creaminess from reduced-fat cream cheese. If you prefer, you may substitute cream cheese flavored with chives and onions for the fresh chives and chopped onions in the ingredient list.

3 POUNDS PEELED YUKON GOLD POTATOES, QUARTERED
⅔ CUP FAT-FREE MILK
1 TEASPOON SALT
⅔ CUP ⅓-LESS-FAT CREAM CHEESE
2 TABLESPOONS FRESH CHIVES
1 TABLESPOON CHOPPED ONION

1. Place the potatoes in a Dutch oven and cover them with water. Bring to a boil; then reduce the heat and simmer for 10 minutes or until tender.
2. Drain the potatoes and return them to the pan. Add the milk and salt.
3. Mash the potatoes with a potato masher.
4. Add the cream cheese, chives, and onion and stir until blended. Serve immediately.

Creamed Spinach

SERVES 4

▸ CALORIES: 130, TOTAL FAT: 4 G, SATURATED FAT: 1 G, FIBER: 4 G,
SODIUM: 170 MG, CHOLESTEROL: 5 MG

Spinach is a nutritional star, with folate, beta-carotene, and other nutrients. However, when the creamed version is loaded with butter, it fails the test. This recipe skips the butter and gets its creaminess from evaporated milk.

2 TEASPOONS EXTRA-VIRGIN OLIVE OIL
2 SHALLOTS, FINELY CHOPPED
4 TEASPOONS FLOUR
1½ CUPS 2 PERCENT MILK
½ CUP LOW-SODIUM CHICKEN BROTH
TWO 10-OUNCE PACKAGES FROZEN SPINACH, THAWED AND DRAINED
2 TABLESPOONS FAT-FREE EVAPORATED MILK
PINCH OF GROUND NUTMEG
SALT AND FRESHLY GROUND BLACK PEPPER

1. In a large pan over medium heat, heat the oil. Add the shallots and cook, stirring, until they are softened, about 2 minutes.
2. Add the flour and cook, stirring, for 30 seconds.
3. Add the milk and broth and bring to a simmer. Cook for 2 minutes, scraping up any browned bits on the bottom of the pan.
4. Add the spinach and simmer until tender, about 5 minutes.
5. Stir in the evaporated milk and nutmeg. Season with salt and pepper, and serve immediately.

Chickpeas with Raisins and Cilantro

SERVES 8

▶ CALORIES: 237, TOTAL FAT: 10 G, SATURATED FAT: 1 G, FIBER: 5 G, SODIUM: 336 MG, CHOLESTEROL: 0 MG

Raisins may be tiny and wrinkled, but don't let their looks fool you: they are crammed with fiber and cancer-fighting antioxidants. The two common varieties are black raisins and golden raisins—they are nearly identical in nutritional value, so use either one.

1 CUP RAISINS
¼ CUP RED WINE VINEGAR
2 TEASPOONS SUGAR
THREE 15.5-OUNCE CANS CHICKPEAS, DRAINED AND RINSED
1 CUP FRESH CILANTRO
4 SCALLIONS, THINLY SLICED
⅓ CUP EXTRA-VIRGIN OLIVE OIL
½ TEASPOON GROUND CUMIN
½ TEASPOON SALT
¼ TEASPOON FRESHLY GROUND BLACK PEPPER

1. In a small saucepan, combine the raisins, vinegar, and sugar. Bring the mixture to a simmer; then remove it from the heat and let it cool.
2. In a large bowl, mix together the chickpeas, cilantro, scallions, and raisin mixture.
3. In a small bowl, combine the oil, cumin, salt, and pepper.
4. Pour the oil mixture over the chickpeas, stir well, and serve.

White Beans with Rosemary and Garlic

SERVES 4

▶ CALORIES: 245, TOTAL FAT: 9 G, SATURATED FAT: 1 G, FIBER: 9 G, SODIUM: 246 MG, CHOLESTEROL: 1 MG

This dish uses canned cannellini beans, but dried ones may also be used by soaking them in water for six hours before cooking. If you can't find cannellini beans, you may also use great northern beans.

2 TABLESPOONS EXTRA-VIRGIN OLIVE OIL

2 GARLIC CLOVES, SMASHED

¼ TEASPOON RED PEPPER FLAKES

1 PLUM TOMATO, CHOPPED

1 SPRIG ROSEMARY

TWO 15.5-OUNCE CANS CANNELLINI BEANS, DRAINED AND RINSED

½ CUP WATER

¼ CUP CHOPPED FRESH PARSLEY

SALT

1 TABLESPOON GRATED PARMESAN

1. Heat 1 tablespoon of the olive oil in a large skillet over medium-high heat. Add the garlic and red pepper flakes and cook for 1 minute.

2. Add the tomato and rosemary and cook for 2 minutes.

3. Add the cannellini beans and cook 5 minutes, partially smashing the beans with the back of a wooden spoon.

4. Remove the rosemary sprig and stir in the water and parsley. Season with salt and sprinkle with Parmesan.

5. Turn on the broiler and place the pan in the broiler. Broil until the beans are golden on top.

6. Remove the beans from the oven, drizzle them with the remaining tablespoon of olive oil, and serve.

Baked Beans 'n' Greens

SERVES 6

▶ CALORIES: 393, TOTAL FAT: 4 G, SATURATED FAT: 1 G, FIBER: 18 G, SODIUM: 678 MG, CHOLESTEROL: 7 MG

Classic baked beans are a staple at every summer barbecue, but they may be high in sugar and nutritionally don't offer much besides fiber. This version gets a boost from leafy greens, which are high in antioxidants and calcium.

1 TABLESPOON EXTRA-VIRGIN OLIVE OIL

½ ONION, CHOPPED

1 CELERY STALK, FINELY CHOPPED

1 CARROT, PEELED AND FINELY CHOPPED

1 GARLIC CLOVE, FINELY CHOPPED

¼ TEASPOON SALT, PLUS MORE FOR SEASONING

¼ TEASPOON FRESHLY GROUND BLACK PEPPER

1 BUNCH SWISS CHARD OR MUSTARD GREENS, STEMMED
   AND LEAVES CHOPPED

½ CUP DICED SMOKED TURKEY (ABOUT 2 OUNCES)

¼ CUP WATER

ONE 15-OUNCE CAN WHOLE TOMATOES, CRUSHED BY HAND

TWO 15-OUNCE CANS LOW-SODIUM PINTO BEANS, DRAINED AND RINSED

ONE 15-OUNCE CAN NAVY BEANS, UNDRAINED

¼ CUP CHOPPED FRESH PARSLEY

1 TEASPOON CHOPPED FRESH THYME

1 TEASPOON CHOPPED FRESH OREGANO

1. Preheat the oven to 375°F.

2. Heat the oil in a large skillet over medium heat. Add the onion, celery, carrot, garlic, salt, and pepper. Cook, stirring occasionally, until the vegetables are soft, about 7 minutes.

3. Add the Swiss chard, turkey, and water to the skillet. Cook, stirring, until the chard wilts slightly, about 3 minutes.

continued ▶

4. Add the tomatoes with their juice, increase the heat to medium-high, and simmer until the liquid is slightly reduced, about 5 minutes.

5. Add the pinto beans and navy beans with their liquid. Add the parsley, thyme, and oregano, and return the beans to a simmer.

6. Use a potato masher or fork to coarsely mash some of the beans. Season with salt.

7. Transfer the beans to a 2-quart baking dish; cover and bake for 45 minutes.

8. Uncover and bake for 10 more minutes before serving.

Quinoa with Lemon and Fresh Herbs

SERVES 4

▸ CALORIES: 391, TOTAL FAT: 18 G, SATURATED FAT: 3 G, FIBER: 5 G, SODIUM: 176 MG, CHOLESTEROL: 0 MG

Quinoa is packed with protein, fiber, and iron. Note that it should always be rinsed well before use; quinoa has a soapy-tasting coating that washes away when rinsed. The best tool to use for this is a fine-mesh strainer.

2¾ CUPS LOW-SODIUM CHICKEN STOCK
½ CUP FRESH LEMON JUICE
1½ CUPS QUINOA
¼ CUP EXTRA-VIRGIN OLIVE OIL
¾ CUP CHOPPED FRESH BASIL LEAVES
¼ CUP CHOPPED FRESH PARSLEY LEAVES
1 TABLESPOON CHOPPED FRESH THYME LEAVES
2 TEASPOONS LEMON ZEST
SALT AND FRESHLY GROUND BLACK PEPPER

1. In a medium saucepan, combine the chicken stock, ¼ cup of lemon juice, and quinoa. Bring to a boil over medium-high heat. Reduce the heat to low, cover the pan, and simmer until the liquid is absorbed, 12 to 15 minutes.
2. In a small bowl, mix together the olive oil, the remaining ¼ cup of lemon juice, basil, parsley, thyme, and lemon zest. Season with salt and pepper. Pour the dressing over the quinoa, toss until well blended, and serve.

Couscous with Squash, Zucchini, and Dried Cranberries

SERVES 6

▸ CALORIES: 253, TOTAL FAT: 5 G, SATURATED FAT: 1 G, FIBER: 4 G, SODIUM: 318 MG, CHOLESTEROL: 0 MG

Couscous, which is a fast-cooking pasta made from wheat, also gains flavor from sauces and, here, from fruits and vegetables. Dried cranberries add sweetness to the late-summer vegetables.

2 TABLESPOONS EXTRA-VIRGIN OLIVE OIL
½ RED ONION, CHOPPED
1 YELLOW SQUASH, THINLY SLICED
1 ZUCCHINI, THINLY SLICED
SALT AND FRESHLY GROUND PEPPER
½ CUP DRIED CRANBERRIES
2 CUPS LOW-SODIUM CHICKEN BROTH
1½ CUPS COUSCOUS

1. Heat the oil in a large, high-sided skillet over medium-high heat, and add the onion, squash, and zucchini. Sauté until tender, about 5 minutes. Season with salt and pepper.
2. Add the cranberries and broth and bring to a boil.
3. Stir in the couscous; cover, turn off the heat, and let it sit for 10 minutes.
4. Remove the lid, fluff the couscous with a fork, and serve.

Broccolini with Leeks and Bacon

SERVES 8

▶ CALORIES: 81, TOTAL FAT: 3 G, SATURATED FAT: 1 G, FIBER: 2 G, SODIUM: 216 MG, CHOLESTEROL: 4 MG

Broccolini resembles broccoli but has smaller florets and much longer and thinner stems that are completely edible. Like regular broccoli, broccolini is an excellent source of vitamins A, C, and K. This dish gets a flavor boost from center-cut bacon, which has less fat than regular bacon.

4 SLICES CENTER-CUT BACON

1 POUND BROCCOLINI, TRIMMED AND HALVED

2 LEEKS, HALVED LENGTHWISE AND CUT INTO 2-INCH PIECES

¼ TEASPOON DRIED OREGANO

¼ TEASPOON CRUSHED RED PEPPER

4 GARLIC CLOVES, THINLY SLICED

¼ CUP LOW-SODIUM CHICKEN BROTH

1½ TABLESPOONS BALSAMIC VINEGAR

¾ TEASPOONS SALT

1. In a large nonstick skillet over medium-high heat, cook the bacon until crisp.
2. Remove the bacon from the pan and discard all but 2 teaspoons of the pan drippings. Drain the bacon on a paper-towel-lined plate. When cool enough to handle, crumble it and set aside.
3. Add the broccolini and leeks to the pan with the bacon drippings, and sauté for 4 minutes.
4. Add the oregano, red pepper, and garlic, and sauté for 3 minutes.
5. Stir in chicken broth, vinegar, and salt, and cook for 30 seconds or until the liquid is almost evaporated.
6. Sprinkle the broccolini and leeks with the crumbled bacon and serve.

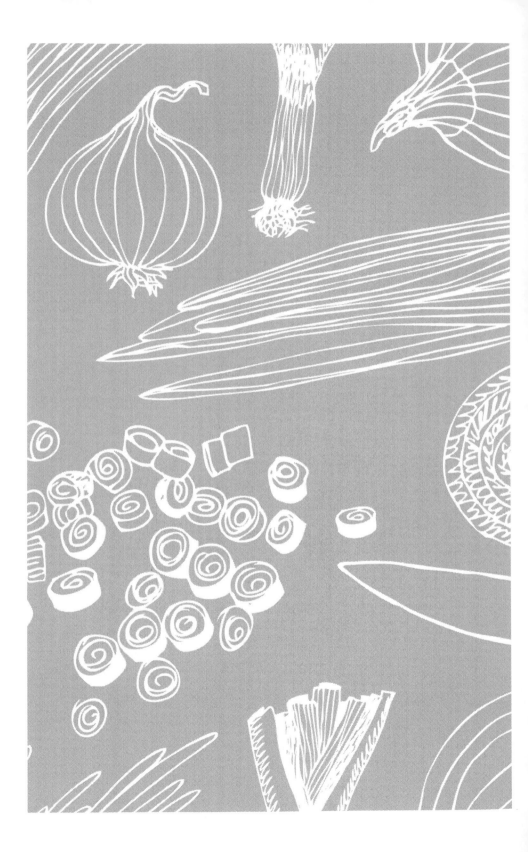

CHAPTER TEN

Entrées

Eggplant Curry with Basil and Chickpeas

Black Beans and Rice

Acorn Squash with Tofu-Spinach Stuffing and Pita Salad

Curried Butternut Squash with Couscous and Chutney

Linguine with Goat Cheese and Zucchini

Vegetarian Club Sandwich with White Beans and Avocado

Soft Tacos with Mushrooms and Swiss Chard

Beefless Sloppy Joes

Halibut with Citrus, Tomatoes, and Olives

Halibut with Sweet Potato and Lentils

Tuna with Mojo Sauce

Tuna Noodle Casserole

Grilled Snapper with Olives and White Wine Sauce

Lemon-Basil Spaghetti with Salmon

Coconut Fish Sticks with Yogurt Dipping Sauce

Seared Scallops with Mango Salsa

Salmon Burgers with Homemade Pickles

Shepherd's Pie

Classic Meatloaf with Ground Chicken

Beef Stir-Fry with Mushrooms and Swiss Chard

Eggplant Curry with Basil and Chickpeas

SERVES 4

▶ CALORIES: 339, TOTAL FAT: 5 G, SATURATED FAT: 1 G, FIBER: 11 G, SODIUM: 697 MG, CHOLESTEROL: 0 MG

If you only know eggplant as a stand-in for chicken in eggplant Parmesan, you need to become better acquainted with it. The purple vegetable is very low in calories and has potassium, folate, magnesium, fiber, and vitamins. It also has a meaty texture, making it a great replacement for meat in vegetarian dishes like this curry.

1 CUP BROWN RICE

1 TABLESPOON EXTRA-VIRGIN OLIVE OIL

1 ONION, CHOPPED

2 PINTS CHERRY TOMATOES, HALVED

1 EGGPLANT, CUT INTO ½-INCH PIECES

1½ TEASPOONS CURRY POWDER

1 TEASPOON SALT

¼ TEASPOON FRESHLY GROUND BLACK PEPPER

2 CUPS WATER

ONE 15.5-OUNCE CAN CHICKPEAS, RINSED

½ CUP FRESH BASIL

1. Cook the rice according to the package directions.
2. Heat the oil in a large saucepan over medium-high heat. Add the onion and cook, stirring occasionally, until softened, 4 to 6 minutes.
3. Stir in the tomatoes, eggplant, curry powder, salt, and pepper. Cook, stirring, until fragrant, about 2 minutes.
4. Add the water to the saucepan and bring to a boil. Reduce the heat and simmer, partially covered, until the eggplant is tender, 12 to 15 minutes.
5. Stir in the chickpeas and cook until heated through, about 3 minutes.
6. Remove the saucepan from heat and stir in the basil. Serve with the rice.

Black Beans and Rice

SERVES 4

▶ CALORIES: 368, TOTAL FAT: 5 G, SATURATED FAT: 1 G, FIBER: 11 G, SODIUM: 777 MG, CHOLESTEROL: 0 MG

This may sound like a side, but this dish actually makes a delicious light lunch when topped with avocado and salsa and served with whole-grain tortilla chips. Black beans are high in protein, but you can boost that amount even more by adding grilled fish or chicken.

1 CUP BROWN RICE

1 TABLESPOON EXTRA-VIRGIN OLIVE OIL

1 ONION, CHOPPED

1 BELL PEPPER, SEEDED AND CUT INTO ¼-INCH PIECES

2 GARLIC CLOVES, CHOPPED

1 TEASPOON SALT

¼ TEASPOON FRESHLY GROUND BLACK PEPPER

1 TEASPOON GROUND CUMIN

TWO 15.5-OUNCE CANS LOW-SODIUM BLACK BEANS,
    DRAINED AND RINSED

1 TEASPOON DRIED OREGANO

1 CUP WATER

1 TABLESPOON RED WINE VINEGAR

4 RADISHES, CUT INTO ½-INCH PIECES

¼ CUP FRESH CILANTRO

1. Cook the rice according to the package directions.

2. Heat the oil in a large saucepan over medium-high heat. Add the onion, bell pepper, garlic, salt, and black pepper. Cook, stirring occasionally, until the onion and bell pepper are softened, 5 to 7 minutes.

3. Stir in the cumin and cook for 1 minute.

4. Add the beans, oregano, and water. Cover and simmer for 10 minutes.

5. Add the vinegar. Thicken the mixture by mashing some of the beans in the saucepan with the back of a fork.

6. Serve with the rice and top with the radishes and cilantro.

Acorn Squash with Tofu-Spinach Stuffing and Pita Salad

SERVES 4

▶ CALORIES: 396, TOTAL FAT: 19 G, SATURATED FAT: 3 G, FIBER: 9 G, SODIUM: 491 MG, CHOLESTEROL: 5 MG

Acorn squash is a round, green winter variety that is full of fiber—9 grams in just one cup—and vitamin C. In this dish, be sure to use firm tofu in the stuffing for the best results.

2 ACORN SQUASH, HALVED, STEMMED, AND SEEDED

4 TABLESPOONS CHOPPED FRESH DILL

¼ TEASPOON SALT, PLUS MORE FOR SEASONING

FRESHLY GROUND BLACK PEPPER

3 TABLESPOONS EXTRA-VIRGIN OLIVE OIL

1 RED ONION, CUT INTO ½-INCH PIECES

3 GARLIC CLOVES, MINCED

ONE 14-OUNCE PACKAGE FIRM TOFU, DRAINED AND
    COARSELY CRUMBLED

1 PINT CHERRY TOMATOES, HALVED

ONE 5-OUNCE PACKAGE BABY SPINACH

2 TABLESPOONS SHREDDED PARMESAN CHEESE

3 TEASPOONS FRESH LEMON JUICE

2 WHOLE-WHEAT PITAS, TOASTED AND TORN INTO 1-INCH PIECES

1. Place the squash in a large, microwave-safe bowl. Add 1 tablespoon of the dill, a splash of water, and season with salt and pepper. Cover with plastic wrap, pierce the plastic with a fork, and microwave for 15 minutes or until tender.

2. Heat 1 tablespoon of the oil in a large nonstick skillet over medium heat. Add the onion and garlic, and cook, stirring, for 3 minutes, until the onion is soft.

3. Stir in the tofu and ¼ teaspoon of salt. Cook without stirring for 2 minutes; then cook 3 minutes while stirring constantly until the tofu is browned.

4. Push the tofu and onion mixture to one side of the pan. Add half of the tomatoes to the other side and season with salt. Cook, stirring the tomatoes, for 3 minutes, then stir them into the tofu and onion mixture.

5. Add half of the spinach and a splash of water, and stir until the spinach wilts.

6. Stir in 1 tablespoon of the Parmesan and 1 teaspoon of the lemon juice. In a large bowl, toss the pitas, the remaining spinach, the remaining tomatoes, the remaining 3 tablespoons of dill, the remaining tablespoon of Parmesan, the remaining 2 tablespoons of olive oil, and the remaining 2 teaspoons of lemon juice, and season with salt.

7. Spoon the tofu mixture into the squash. Serve with the pita salad.

Curried Butternut Squash with Couscous and Chutney

SERVES 6

▸ CALORIES: 510, TOTAL FAT: 18 G, SATURATED FAT: 6 G, FIBER: 8 G, SODIUM: 528 MG, CHOLESTEROL: 27 MG

Chutney is a sweet Indian condiment that is a good foil for the savory taste of curries. One of the most common chutneys is made with mango. Its jam-like consistency makes it also delicious as a dip for spicy hors d'oeuvres.

2 TABLESPOONS VEGETABLE OIL
1 ONION, CUT INTO ½-INCH HALF-MOONS
2 GARLIC CLOVES, MINCED
1 BUTTERNUT SQUASH, PEELED, SEEDED, AND DICED
1 TABLESPOON CURRY POWDER
1½ TEASPOONS PLUS ½ TEASPOON SALT
2 CUPS LOW-SODIUM VEGETABLE BROTH
½ CUP HEAVY CREAM
2 CUPS WATER
2 CUPS INSTANT COUSCOUS
½ CUP CHOPPED PEANUTS, FOR GARNISH
½ CUP COMMERCIAL CHUTNEY, FOR GARNISH

1. Heat the oil in a large skillet over medium heat. Add the onion and garlic, and cook, stirring occasionally, until softened, 5 to 7 minutes.
2. Add the squash, curry powder, and 1½ teaspoons salt. Stir well. Add the broth and bring to a boil.
3. Reduce heat to medium-low, cover, and simmer until the squash is cooked through and most of the liquid has evaporated, 15 to 20 minutes.
4. Stir in the cream and cook, uncovered, over medium-high heat until the sauce has thickened, 3 to 5 minutes.
5. Meanwhile, bring the water and ½ teaspoon of salt to a boil. Place the couscous in a large bowl and pour the boiling water over it. Cover and let stand for 5 to 7 minutes or until all water is absorbed. Fluff the couscous with a fork.
6. Serve the squash over the couscous, garnished with peanuts and chutney.

Linguine with Goat Cheese and Zucchini

SERVES 4

▶ CALORIES: 455, TOTAL FAT: 12 G, SATURATED FAT: 6 G, FIBER: 4 G, SODIUM: 746 MG, CHOLESTEROL: 16 MG

Goat cheese is lower in fat and calories than many hard cheeses. And because it's so soft, it melts beautifully into a creamy sauce, like in this pasta dish.

12 OUNCES WHOLE-WHEAT LINGUINE
1 TABLESPOON EXTRA-VIRGIN OLIVE OIL
1 POUND ZUCCHINI, CUT INTO THIN HALF-MOONS
1¼ TEASPOONS SALT
½ TEASPOON FRESHLY GROUND BLACK PEPPER
1 GARLIC CLOVE, CHOPPED
5 OUNCES GOAT CHEESE
2 TEASPOONS GRATED LEMON ZEST

1. Cook the linguine according to the package directions. Drain the pasta, reserving 1 cup of the pasta water, and return the linguine to the pot.
2. Meanwhile, heat the oil in a medium skillet over medium-high heat. Add the zucchini, ½ teaspoon of salt, and ¼ teaspoon of pepper. Cook, stirring, until the zucchini is tender and any liquid has evaporated, about 5 minutes.
3. Stir in the garlic and cook for 1 minute.
4. Add all but 2 tablespoons of the cheese to the linguine in the pot. Add the reserved pasta water, the remaining ¾ teaspoon of salt, and the remaining ¼ teaspoon of pepper to the linguine. Stir until creamy.
5. Serve the linguine topped with the zucchini, lemon zest, and the remaining 2 tablespoons of cheese.

Vegetarian Club Sandwich with White Beans and Avocado

SERVES 4

▶ CALORIES: 684, TOTAL FAT: 23 G, SATURATED FAT: 3 G, FIBER: 27 G, SODIUM: 464 MG, CHOLESTEROL: 0 MG

Club sandwiches usually contain bacon, mayonnaise, and other meats and cheese—not ideal for someone on a low-cholesterol diet. This version is as satisfying as the real thing but uses creamy white beans as a spread and lots of vegetables for crunch.

TWO 15-OUNCE CANS OF WHITE BEANS, RINSED AND DRAINED

2 TABLESPOONS EXTRA-VIRGIN OLIVE OIL

½ TEASPOON SALT

¼ TEASPOON BLACK FRESHLY GROUND PEPPER

12 SLICES MULTIGRAIN BREAD

1 RED ONION, THINLY SLICED

1 CUCUMBER, THINLY SLICED

ONE 4-OUNCE CONTAINER SPROUTS (ALFALFA, RADISH, BROCCOLI, OR ANY MIX)

2 AVOCADOS, PEELED, PITTED, AND THINLY SLICED

1. In a medium bowl, combine the beans, oil, salt, and pepper. Mash the beans with a fork.
2. Place 8 slices of bread on a work surface. Divide the mashed beans among them; top each with the onion, cucumber, sprouts, and avocado.
3. Stack one open-faced sandwich on top of another until you have four double-decker sandwiches. Top each sandwich with remaining 4 slices of bread; plate and enjoy.

Soft Tacos with Mushrooms and Swiss Chard

SERVES 4

▸ CALORIES: 270, TOTAL FAT: 2 G, SATURATED FAT: 0 G, FIBER: 12 G, SODIUM: 240 MG, CHOLESTEROL: 0 MG

Mushrooms, greens, and beans make a healthful, nutritious filling for corn tortillas. Opt for soft tortillas over crispy shells to save on fat and calories.

½ CUP WATER

2 YELLOW ONIONS, THINLY SLICED

1 TEASPOON REDUCED-SODIUM TAMARI

8 OUNCES SLICED BUTTON MUSHROOMS

1 BUNCH SWISS CHARD, STEMS AND LEAVES SEPARATED AND BOTH
    THINLY SLICED

ONE 15-OUNCE CAN PINTO BEANS, RINSED AND DRAINED

8 CORN TORTILLAS

1 RED BELL PEPPER, SEEDED AND CHOPPED

1. Bring the water to a simmer in a deep skillet over medium-high heat. Add the onions and cook for 8 minutes, stirring occasionally, until they begin to soften and brown.

2. Add the tamari, mushrooms, and Swiss chard stems and reduce the heat to medium. Cover and cook for 15 minutes or until the mushrooms are tender, stirring frequently and adding 1 or 2 tablespoons of water if the onions begin to stick.

3. Stir in the Swiss chard leaves and beans, cover, and cook for 5 minutes or until the leaves wilt.

4. Warm the tortillas, fill them with the bean mixture, and serve topped with the red bell pepper.

Beefless Sloppy Joes

SERVES 6

▶ CALORIES: 257, TOTAL FAT: 9 G, SATURATED FAT: 1 G, FIBER: 6 G, SODIUM: 486 MG, CHOLESTEROL: 0 MG

Sloppy Joe sandwiches are traditionally made with ground beef, which may make them high in saturated fat. This version substitutes mushrooms instead, meaning you get all the flavor without harming your heart.

1 POUND CREMINI MUSHROOMS, HALVED

1 TABLESPOON EXTRA-VIRGIN OLIVE OIL

1 LARGE SWEET ONION, DICED

1½ CUPS PLUS 4 TABLESPOONS LIGHT BEER

¼ TEASPOON SALT, PLUS MORE FOR SEASONING

⅓ CUP FINELY CHOPPED WALNUTS

1 GREEN PEPPER, DICED

¾ TEASPOON FRESHLY GROUND BLACK PEPPER

½ TEASPOON CHIPOTLE CHILI POWDER

¼ CUP KETCHUP

3 TABLESPOONS TOMATO PASTE

6 WHOLE-WHEAT HAMBURGER BUNS

1. Pulse the mushrooms in batches in a food processor until they are finely chopped.
2. Heat the oil in a large nonstick skillet over medium-high heat. Add the onion, 1 tablespoon of the beer, and salt, and cook, stirring frequently, until the onion is lightly browned, about 5 minutes.
3. Add the walnuts and green pepper, and cook, stirring occasionally, for 3 minutes.
4. Add the mushrooms, black pepper, and chipotle chili powder. Cook, stirring frequently, for about 5 minutes or until mushrooms are just cooked through.
5. Add the remaining beer, the ketchup, tomato paste, and a large pinch of salt. Cook while stirring until the sauce is a fairly thick consistency, about 2 minutes.
6. Spoon the mixture onto the buns and serve.

Halibut with Citrus, Tomatoes, and Olives

SERVES 4

▸ CALORIES: 339, TOTAL FAT: 12 G, SATURATED FAT: 1 G, FIBER: 5 G, SODIUM: 602 MG, CHOLESTEROL: 54 MG

Halibut has a sweeter flavor than other fish, and firm, white flesh. If you can't find it in the seafood section, cod and haddock will both work well.

1 TABLESPOON EXTRA-VIRGIN OLIVE OIL, DIVIDED
1 YELLOW ONION, THINLY SLICED
1 CUP GREEN OLIVES, PITTED AND HALVED
2 ORANGES, PEELED, SEPARATED INTO SEGMENTS,
    AND MEMBRANES REMOVED
ONE 28-OUNCE CAN DICED TOMATOES, UNDRAINED
¼ TEASPOON SALT
¼ TEASPOON BLACK PEPPER
1½ POUNDS HALIBUT, SKIN REMOVED, CUT INTO 2-INCH PIECES
¼ CUP FRESH DILL, CHOPPED

1. Heat the oil in a large saucepan over medium heat. Add the onion and cook until it is soft, about 5 minutes.
2. Add the olives, orange segments, and tomatoes. Cover and simmer for 10 minutes. Add the salt and pepper.
3. Place the fish in the pan and spoon the sauce over it. Cover and simmer until the fish is cooked through, about 7 minutes.
4. Divide the fish and sauce among four plates, sprinkle with dill, and serve.

Halibut with Sweet Potato and Lentils

SERVES 4

▶ CALORIES: 529, TOTAL FAT: 13 G, SATURATED FAT: 2 G, FIBER: 11 G, SODIUM: 691 MG, CHOLESTEROL: 61 MG

Lentils, rich in folic acid, fiber, and vitamins, belong in everyone's diet, and they are also an economical source of protein without cholesterol. Their different varieties—brown, green, and red—are relatively interchangeable, although brown and red lentils have a shorter cooking time.

2 TABLESPOONS EXTRA-VIRGIN OLIVE OIL, DIVIDED

1 ONION, CHOPPED

2 GARLIC CLOVES, CHOPPED

1 SWEET POTATO, PEELED AND CUT INTO ¼-INCH PIECES

2½ CUPS LOW-SODIUM CHICKEN BROTH

1¼ CUPS GREEN LENTILS, RINSED

SALT AND FRESHLY GROUND BLACK PEPPER

FOUR 6-OUNCE PIECES OF HALIBUT FILLET

¼ CUP DIJON MUSTARD

¼ CUP DRY WHITE WINE

1 TABLESPOON CHOPPED FRESH TARRAGON

1. Heat 1 tablespoon of the olive oil in a large saucepan over medium heat. Add the onion and cook, stirring occasionally, until soft, 5 to 6 minutes.

2. Add the garlic and sweet potato, and cook, stirring, for 1 minute.

3. Add the broth and lentils, and simmer, covered, until lentils are tender, 20 to 25 minutes. Season with salt and pepper.

4. Meanwhile, heat the remaining tablespoon of oil in a skillet over medium-high heat. Season the fish with salt and pepper and cook in the skillet until opaque throughout, 3 to 5 minutes per side.

5. In a small bowl, whisk together the mustard, wine, and tarragon.

6. Serve the fish over the lentils and drizzled with the sauce.

Tuna with Mojo Sauce

SERVES 4

▸ CALORIES: 287, TOTAL FAT: 22 G, SATURATED FAT: 4 G, FIBER: 0 G, SODIUM: 754 MG, CHOLESTEROL: 32 MG

Mojo is a citrus-based sauce made with garlic, olive oil, and fresh herbs. It goes perfectly with tuna steaks, which may be served medium-rare. To cook them medium-well done, increase the grilling time to four to six minutes per side.

4 GARLIC CLOVES, CHOPPED
5 TABLESPOONS EXTRA-VIRGIN OLIVE OIL
1 FRESH JALAPEÑO, SEEDED AND THINLY SLICED
JUICE OF 4 LIMES
⅓ CUP FRESH CILANTRO, COARSELY CHOPPED
1 TEASPOON SALT, PLUS MORE FOR SEASONING
FRESHLY GROUND BLACK PEPPER
TWO 12-OUNCE TUNA STEAKS, ABOUT 1¼-INCH THICK

1. Heat an outdoor grill or indoor grill pan to medium-high.
2. In a medium microwave-safe bowl, stir together the garlic and 4 tablespoons of olive oil. Cover it loosely with plastic wrap and microwave it until the garlic is soft and aromatic, about 2 minutes.
3. Stir in the jalapeño, lime juice, cilantro, and salt. Set aside to cool.
4. Brush the tuna with the remaining tablespoon of olive oil and season with salt and pepper.
5. Grill the tuna, turning once, until the fish has grill marks on its surface, 3 to 5 minutes per side for medium rare. Let rest for 5 minutes.
6. Slice each tuna steak in half and serve drizzled with the mojo.

Tuna Noodle Casserole

SERVES 6

▸ CALORIES: 476, TOTAL FAT: 7 G, SATURATED FAT: 1 G, FIBER: 11 G, SODIUM: 733 MG, CHOLESTEROL: 66 MG

This dish is often made with egg noodles and high-fat cream of mushroom soup. While delicious, it isn't necessarily heart-healthful. This recipe does things differently by using fresh mushrooms, 2 percent milk, broccoli, and whole-wheat noodles.

½ POUND WHOLE-WHEAT FETTUCCINE, BROKEN INTO THIRDS

5 SLICES WHOLE-WHEAT BREAD

1 TABLESPOON ORGANIC CANOLA OIL

1 CUP CHOPPED ONION

1 CELERY STALK, FINELY DICED

ONE 10-OUNCE BOX WHITE MUSHROOMS, STEMMED AND CHOPPED

¼ CUP FLOUR

3 CUPS 2 PERCENT MILK

1 CUP LOW-SODIUM CHICKEN BROTH

¼ TEASPOON GROUND BLACK PEPPER

ONE 10-OUNCE BOX FROZEN CHOPPED BROCCOLI, THAWED

ONE 10-OUNCE BOX FROZEN PEAS, THAWED

FOUR 6-OUNCE CANS CHUNK LIGHT TUNA IN WATER, DRAINED

1. Preheat the oven to 425°F.

2. Bring a pot of water to a boil and cook the fettuccine according to the package directions. Drain and set aside.

3. Place the bread in a food processor and pulse for 30 seconds until it becomes breadcrumbs.

4. Heat the oil in a large skillet over medium heat. Add the onion and cook, stirring, until translucent, about 5 minutes.

5. Add the celery and cook, stirring, until just tender, about 6 minutes.

6. Add the mushrooms and cook, stirring, until they release their liquid, 5 to 7 minutes.

7. Add the flour and stir vigorously with a wooden spoon until there are no lumps.

8. Add the milk and broth, stir to combine, and bring the mixture to a boil, stirring frequently.

9. Reduce the heat to a vigorous simmer and cook, stirring, until the liquid thickens and reduces by about ½ cup, 7 to 8 minutes.

10. Add the pepper and stir to combine.

11. In a large bowl, combine the fettuccine, vegetable and mushroom mixture, broccoli, peas, and tuna.

12. Pour the ingredients into a 9-by-13-inch casserole. Top with the breadcrumbs and bake for 25 minutes or until the top is golden and toasted. Serve hot.

Grilled Snapper with Olives and White Wine Sauce

SERVES 4

▶ CALORIES: 279, TOTAL FAT: 10 G, SATURATED FAT: 2 G, FIBER: 2 G, SODIUM: 468 MG, CHOLESTEROL: 63 MG

When choosing a white wine for this dish, a dry white is best, such as Sauvignon Blanc, Chardonnay, or Pinot Grigio.

FOUR 6-OUNCE SNAPPER FILLETS
2 TABLESPOONS EXTRA-VIRGIN OLIVE OIL, PLUS MORE FOR THE FISH
SALT AND FRESHLY GROUND BLACK PEPPER
1 ONION, FINELY SLICED
2 GARLIC CLOVES, FINELY CHOPPED
¼ CUP DRY WHITE WINE
2 TOMATOES, CHOPPED
¼ CUP GREEN OLIVES, PITTED AND CHOPPED
2 TABLESPOONS CAPERS
1 SERRANO PEPPER, FINELY CHOPPED
½ TEASPOON SUGAR
1 BAY LEAF

1. Heat the grill to high.
2. Brush the snapper with some oil and season with salt and pepper. Grill for 2 minutes per side, remove from the grill, and cover to keep warm.
3. Heat the oil in a medium skillet over medium-high heat. Add the onions and garlic, and cook until soft, 5 to 7 minutes.
4. Add the wine and cook for 3 to 5 minutes or until slightly reduced.
5. Add the tomatoes, olives, capers, serrano pepper, sugar, and bay leaf. Bring the sauce to a boil and cook until thickened.
6. Reduce the heat, add the fish, and cook for 2 minutes or until the fish is completely cooked through.
7. Spoon the fish fillets onto four plates and serve each with the olives and sauce.

Lemon-Basil Spaghetti with Salmon

SERVES 4

▶ CALORIES: 462, TOTAL FAT: 18 G, SATURATED FAT: 3 G, FIBER: 8 G, SODIUM: 573 MG, CHOLESTEROL: 66 MG

Like tuna, salmon is another fish that may be served successfully anywhere between medium-rare to well-done. If you like salmon medium-rare, cook it for two minutes per side.

½ POUND WHOLE-WHEAT SPAGHETTI

1 GARLIC CLOVE, MINCED

3 TABLESPOONS EXTRA-VIRGIN OLIVE OIL

½ TEASPOON SALT, PLUS MORE FOR SEASONING

½ TEASPOON FRESHLY GROUND BLACK PEPPER,
    PLUS MORE FOR SEASONING

FOUR 4-OUNCE SALMON FILLETS

¼ CUP CHOPPED FRESH BASIL LEAVES

3 TABLESPOONS CAPERS

ZEST OF 1 LEMON

2 TABLESPOONS LEMON JUICE

2 CUPS BABY SPINACH

1. Bring a large pot of water to a boil. Add the spaghetti and cook until al dente, stirring occasionally, 8 to 10 minutes. Drain and transfer the spaghetti to a large bowl.

2. Add the garlic, 2 tablespoons of olive oil, ½ teaspoon of salt, and ½ teaspoon of pepper, and toss to combine.

3. Heat the remaining tablespoon of olive oil in a medium skillet over medium-high heat.

continued ▶

4. Season the salmon fillets with salt and pepper, and cook them to the desired degree of doneness. Remove the salmon from the pan.

5. Add the basil, capers, lemon zest, and lemon juice to the spaghetti and toss to combine.

6. Place ½ cup of spinach each into four shallow bowls. Divide the spaghetti among the bowls and serve topped with a piece of salmon.

Coconut Fish Sticks with Yogurt Dipping Sauce

SERVES 6

▶ CALORIES: 206, TOTAL FAT: 5 G, SATURATED FAT: 3 G, FIBER: 2 G, SODIUM: 253 MG, CHOLESTEROL: 58 MG

This kid-friendly recipe makes eating fish fun by coating it in a crunchy coconut-breadcrumb mixture. The fish sticks may also be frozen on a baking sheet uncooked and stored for up to one month in the freezer. Bake them directly from the freezer for 20 to 25 minutes.

For the fish sticks:
COOKING SPRAY
1½ POUNDS TILAPIA FILLETS
1¼ CUPS WHOLE-WHEAT BREADCRUMBS
⅓ CUP SWEETENED SHREDDED COCONUT
2 TABLESPOONS YELLOW CORNMEAL
1 TEASPOON MILD CURRY POWDER
½ TEASPOON SALT, PLUS MORE FOR SEASONING
1 FREE-RANGE OR OMEGA-3 EGG WHITE
1 TABLESPOON WATER

For the yogurt dipping sauce:
⅓ CUP 2 PERCENT GREEK YOGURT
1 CARROT, PEELED AND FINELY GRATED
2 TEASPOONS SWEET CHILI SAUCE
1 TEASPOON LOW-SODIUM SOY SAUCE
1 SCALLION, FINELY CHOPPED
JUICE OF ½ LIME
1 TABLESPOON WATER

continued ▶

To make the fish sticks:

1. Preheat the oven to 425°F.
2. Place a baking rack in a baking pan and spray it with cooking spray.
3. Cut the fish into sticks about 3 inches long and ½-inch thick.
4. In a food processor, combine the breadcrumbs, coconut, cornmeal, curry powder, and salt. Pulse until the coconut is coarsely chopped. Transfer the mixture to a shallow dish.
5. In a separate shallow dish, whisk together the egg white and water.
6. Dip each fish stick first into the egg white, shaking off the excess, and then coat each fish stick thoroughly with the breadcrumb mixture.
7. Spray the fish sticks with cooking spray, arrange them on the baking rack, and bake them for 15 to 20 minutes, turning them halfway through. Bake them until golden, crispy, and cooked through. Season with salt.

To make the yogurt dipping sauce:

1. Combine the yogurt, carrot, chili sauce, soy sauce, scallion, lime juice, and water in a medium bowl. Season with salt.
2. Cover and refrigerate until serving. Serve alongside the hot fish sticks.

Seared Scallops with Mango Salsa

SERVES 4

▶ CALORIES: 477, TOTAL FAT: 9 G, SATURATED FAT: 1 G, FIBER: 3 G, SODIUM: 518 MG, CHOLESTEROL: 56 MG

This recipe calls for sea scallops, which are larger than bay scallops and are readily available in the supermarket. You might notice a little muscle attached to the scallops. It hangs off to the side like a tag and you can remove it with your fingers.

1 CUP BROWN RICE

2 MANGOES, PITTED AND CUT INTO ½-INCH PIECES

1 CUCUMBER, PEELED AND CUT INTO ½-INCH PIECES

1 TABLESPOON GRATED FRESH GINGER

2 TEASPOONS FRESH LIME JUICE

2 TABLESPOONS EXTRA-VIRGIN OLIVE OIL

½ CUP FRESH CILANTRO, CHOPPED

½ TEASPOON SALT, PLUS MORE FOR SEASONING

FRESHLY GROUND BLACK PEPPER

1½ POUNDS SEA SCALLOPS

1. Cook the rice according to the package directions.
2. In a medium bowl, combine the mangoes, cucumber, ginger, lime juice, 1 tablespoon of olive oil, cilantro, ½ teaspoon of salt, and a large pinch of pepper.
3. Rinse the scallops and pat dry with paper towels. Season them with salt and pepper.
4. Heat the remaining tablespoon of oil in a large skillet over medium-high heat. Add the scallops and cook until cooked through and golden brown, about 2 minutes per side.
5. Serve with the rice and top with salsa.

Salmon Burgers with Homemade Pickles

SERVES 4

▶ CALORIES: 371, TOTAL FAT: 12 G, SATURATED FAT: 3 G, FIBER: 2 G, SODIUM: 652 MG, CHOLESTEROL: 86 MG

This recipe uses raw salmon but if you use canned salmon, the dish is ready in a jiffy because the patties won't have to be completely cooked, only heated through.

¼ CUP RICE VINEGAR

1 TABLESPOON SUGAR

¾ TEASPOON SALT,

1 KIRBY CUCUMBER, VERY THINLY SLICED

¼ WHITE ONION, THINLY SLICED

1¼ POUNDS SKINLESS SALMON FILLET, CUT INTO 1-INCH PIECES

4 SCALLIONS, THINLY SLICED

¼ TEASPOON FRESHLY GROUND BLACK PEPPER

4 WHOLE-WHEAT HAMBURGER BUNS

1. In a medium bowl, combine the vinegar, sugar, and ¼ teaspoon of salt, stirring until everything is dissolved.
2. Add the cucumber and onion, and toss to combine. Let sit, tossing occasionally, for at least 15 minutes and up to 6 hours.
3. Heat the grill to medium-high.
4. In a food processor, pulse the salmon 3 or 4 times just until coarsely chopped.
5. Add the scallions, the remaining ½ teaspoon of salt, and pepper, and pulse to combine.
6. Form the mixture into four ¾-inch-thick patties.
7. Oil the grill grate. Grill the patties, turning once, until opaque, 2 to 4 minutes per side.
8. To serve, place the burgers on buns and top them with the cucumber and onion.

Shepherd's Pie

SERVES 4

▸ CALORIES: 290, TOTAL FAT: 12 G, SATURATED FAT: 4 G, FIBER: 4 G, SODIUM: 370 MG, CHOLESTEROL: 50 MG

Shepherd's pie is one of the classic comfort foods that makes a perfect dinner on a cold winter day. It is usually made with ground beef, but this is a lighter version with ground turkey. And because it calls for red-skinned potatoes, there is no need to peel them.

1 TABLESPOON EXTRA-VIRGIN OLIVE OIL

2 GARLIC CLOVES, MINCED

1 CARROT, PEELED AND FINELY DICED

1 ONION, CHOPPED

8 OUNCES GROUND TURKEY

½ TEASPOON FINELY CHOPPED FRESH THYME

2 TABLESPOONS KETCHUP

1 CUP LOW-SODIUM CHICKEN BROTH

2 TEASPOONS FLOUR

½ CUP FROZEN PEAS, THAWED

¼ TEASPOON SALT, PLUS MORE FOR SEASONING

1 POUND RED-SKINNED POTATOES, CUBED

½ CUP 2 PERCENT MILK, WARMED

⅓ CUP SHREDDED SHARP CHEDDAR CHEESE

1 SCALLION, CHOPPED

FRESHLY GROUND BLACK PEPPER

COOKING SPRAY

1. Preheat the oven to 425°F.

2. Heat the oil in a medium ovenproof skillet over medium-high heat. Add the garlic, carrot, and onion. Cook until they are tender and begin to brown, about 5 minutes.

continued ▸

3. Add the turkey and thyme, and cook, breaking the turkey up with a spoon, until it is cooked through and lightly browned.

4. Stir in the ketchup and cook for 1 minute.

5. In a small bowl, stir the broth and flour together until smooth. Pour the mixture into the skillet and cook until it thickens, about 2 minutes. Stir the peas in and add the salt.

6. Meanwhile, place the potatoes in a medium pot and cover with water. Bring to a boil, lower the heat, and simmer until the potatoes are tender.

7. Drain the potatoes and return them to the pot over low heat. Stir for 2 to 3 minutes to dry them out. Add the milk, cheese, and scallion, and mash the potatoes. Season with salt and pepper.

8. Spoon the mashed potatoes over the meat filling and spread it in an even layer.

9. Lightly mist the potatoes with nonstick cooking spray and bake until they are lightly browned and the filling is bubbling around the edges, 10 to 15 minutes. Serve hot.

Classic Meatloaf with Ground Chicken

SERVES 8

▶ CALORIES: 125, TOTAL FAT: 5 G, SATURATED FAT: 2 G, FIBER: 1 G, SODIUM: 477 MG, CHOLESTEROL: 49 MG

All the flavors of traditional meatloaf are here but with a leaner meat than ground beef. Serve with mashed potatoes or roasted veggies and you have the perfect weeknight dinner.

1 POUND GROUND CHICKEN

½ CUP FINE BREADCRUMBS

1 FREE-RANGE OR OMEGA-3 EGG WHITE

1 CARROT, PEELED AND CUT INTO CHUNKS

1 ONION, CUT INTO CHUNKS

¼ CUP KETCHUP

½ TEASPOON MINCED GARLIC

1 TEASPOON WORCESTERSHIRE SAUCE

¼ TEASPOON CELERY SEED

1 TEASPOON SALT

PINCH OF PEPPER

1. Preheat the oven to 350°F.
2. In a large bowl, combine the chicken, breadcrumbs, and egg white.
3. In a blender combine the carrot, onion, ketchup, garlic, Worcestershire sauce, celery seed, salt, and pepper. Process until the carrot is very fine.
4. Add the vegetable mixture to the meat and mix well with your hands.
5. Form the mixture into a loaf and place it in a lightly greased 9-by-13-inch pan. Cover the loaf with foil and bake for 1 hour.
6. Remove the foil and continue baking the loaf for 15 to 30 minutes, or until meatloaf is cooked through.
7. Slice the loaf into 8 pieces and serve hot.

Beef Stir-Fry with Mushrooms and Swiss Chard

SERVES 4

▶ CALORIES: 300, TOTAL FAT: 15 G, SATURATED FAT: 3 G, FIBER: 2 G, SODIUM: 561 MG, CHOLESTEROL: 41 MG

While beef may be high in cholesterol, using it as an ingredient in a stir-fry instead of as a main course is a good way to enjoy its flavor in a healthier way. This dish combines mushrooms and Swiss chard with the beef, but you may also use broccoli, green beans, and red pepper strips.

1 POUND BONELESS SIRLOIN STEAK, SLICED ¼-INCH THICK

1 TABLESPOON PLUS 2 TEASPOONS CORNSTARCH

1 TABLESPOON PLUS 2 TEASPOONS BALSAMIC VINEGAR

3 TEASPOONS SOY SAUCE

2 TEASPOONS PACKED LIGHT BROWN SUGAR

⅓ CUP WATER

3 TABLESPOONS EXTRA-VIRGIN OLIVE OIL

3 GARLIC CLOVES, THINLY SLICED

½ RED ONION, CUT INTO THIN WEDGES

4 OUNCES MIXED MUSHROOMS, SLICED

1 BUNCH SWISS CHARD, STEMS CUT INTO ½-INCH PIECES
AND LEAVES SHREDDED

¼ TEASPOON SALT

FRESHLY GROUND BLACK PEPPER

JUICE OF ½ LEMON

1. In a medium bowl, combine the beef, 1 tablespoon of cornstarch, 1 tablespoon of vinegar, and 2 teaspoons of soy sauce.

2. In a small bowl, combine the brown sugar, the remaining 2 teaspoons of cornstarch, the remaining 2 teaspoons of vinegar, the remaining 1 teaspoon of soy sauce, and water. Stir until smooth.

3. In a large nonstick skillet over high heat, heat 1 tablespoon of olive oil. Add the beef and cook, stirring occasionally, until just cooked through, 2 to 3 minutes. Transfer to a bowl and wipe out the skillet.

4. Heat the remaining 2 tablespoons of olive oil in the skillet over high heat. Add the garlic and red onion and stir-fry for 2 minutes.

5. Add the mushrooms, Swiss chard stems, and salt. Season with the pepper. Stir-fry until the vegetables are just tender, 4 minutes.

6. Add the Swiss chard leaves and cook until wilted.

7. Stir in the brown sugar mixture and beef. Cook until the sauce thickens, stirring, for about 1 minute.

8. Add the lemon juice and serve.

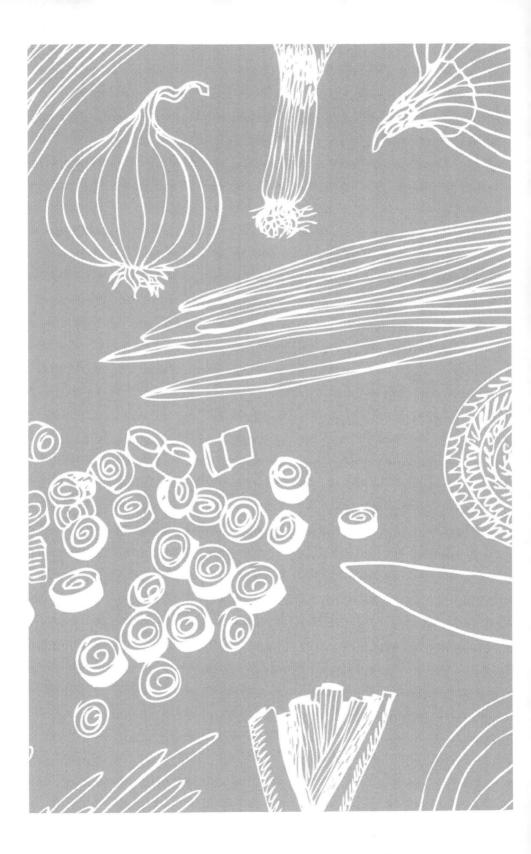

CHAPTER ELEVEN

Desserts

Strawberries with Ricotta Cream and Balsamic Reduction

Blueberries with Lemon Cream

Grilled Plums Topped with Spiced Yogurt

Strawberry Sherbet

Almond-Lemon Cookies

Carrot Cake Cookies

Peanut Butter Cups

Homemade Fudge Pops

Dark Chocolate Pudding

Flourless Chocolate Cake

Strawberries with Ricotta Cream and Balsamic Reduction

SERVES 4

▶ CALORIES: 180, TOTAL FAT: 5 G, SATURATED FAT: 3 G, FIBER: 2 G, SODIUM: 80 MG, CHOLESTEROL: 20 MG

Balsamic vinegar has long been used in Modena, Italy, from where it originates, to enhance the natural flavor of fruit. The type to buy is aged from three to five years and comes in a small bottle. It's a bit expensive, but once you taste these strawberries, you'll be a convert. Think of it as Italy's answer to pure maple syrup.

1 CUP PART-SKIM RICOTTA CHEESE
2 TABLESPOONS HONEY
½ TEASPOON VANILLA EXTRACT
3 TABLESPOONS AGED BALSAMIC VINEGAR
2 TABLESPOONS SUGAR
ONE 16-OUNCE CONTAINER STRAWBERRIES, HULLED AND QUARTERED
2 TABLESPOONS FRESH BASIL LEAVES, CUT INTO RIBBONS

1. Place the ricotta, honey, and vanilla extract in the bowl of a food processor and process until smooth, about 1 minute.
2. Transfer the ricotta to a small bowl and refrigerate for at least 2 hours.
3. In a small saucepan, combine the balsamic vinegar and sugar and bring to a boil. Simmer over medium heat for 2 minutes, stirring occasionally. Allow to cool completely.
4. In a medium bowl, toss the berries with the basil and the balsamic reduction.
5. Serve the ricotta in dessert bowls topped with the strawberries.

Blueberries with Lemon Cream

SERVES 4

▶ CALORIES: 230, TOTAL FAT: 3 G, SATURATED FAT: 0 G, FIBER: 6 G, SODIUM: 35 MG, CHOLESTEROL: 0 MG

Dates are a natural sweetener that replace refined sugar in this dessert. The other surprise ingredient is tofu, which adds creaminess without any taste. If you're having a dinner party, make the lemon cream in advance—it may be refrigerated for up to three days.

2 TABLESPOONS LEMON ZEST
3 TABLESPOONS FRESH LEMON JUICE
8 PITTED DATES, COARSELY CHOPPED
1 TEASPOON VANILLA EXTRACT
⅛ TEASPOON GROUND CARDAMOM
ONE 12-OUNCE PACKAGE SILKEN TOFU, DRAINED
2 CUPS BLUEBERRIES

1. Combine 1 tablespoon of lemon zest, lemon juice, dates, vanilla, cardamom, and tofu in a blender. Purée until smooth.
2. Divide the lemon cream evenly among four bowls; serve with blueberries and the remaining tablespoon of lemon zest.

Grilled Plums Topped with Spiced Yogurt

SERVES 4

▶ CALORIES: 183, TOTAL FAT: 8 G, SATURATED FAT: 1 G, FIBER: 2 G, SODIUM: 25 MG, CHOLESTEROL: 0 MG

Give your grill double duty in the summer by using it to make this light dessert. The sauce may be made in advance and kept covered in the refrigerator until serving time.

For the plums:
6 PLUMS, HALVED AND PITTED
2 TEASPOONS ORGANIC CANOLA OIL
1 TABLESPOON HONEY
PINCH OF GROUND CINNAMON
PINCH OF GRATED ORANGE ZEST

For the spiced yogurt:
1 CUP PLAIN GREEK YOGURT
1 TABLESPOON HONEY
2 TABLESPOONS FRESH ORANGE JUICE
1 TEASPOON GRATED ORANGE ZEST
¼ TEASPOON GROUND CINNAMON
¼ CUP FINELY CHOPPED WALNUTS, TOASTED

To make the plums:

1. Heat the grill to high.
2. Brush the plums with oil on the cut side, drizzle with honey, and sprinkle with cinnamon and orange zest.
3. Place the plums on grill, cut-side down, and grill for 2 minutes or until they start to caramelize and turn golden brown.
4. Turn the plums over and grill until just heated through, about 1 minute.

To make the spiced yogurt:

1. Whisk together the yogurt, honey, orange juice, orange zest, cinnamon, and walnuts in a small bowl.
2. Place 3 plum halves in each dessert bowl and top with the yogurt sauce.

Strawberry Sherbet

SERVES 8

▸ CALORIES: 111, TOTAL FAT: 3 G, SATURATED FAT: 2 G, FIBER: 1 G, SODIUM: 94 MG, CHOLESTEROL: 7 MG

Sherbet is a mix of sorbet, which is dairy-free, and ice cream. This recipe uses fresh strawberries, but you can also use frozen ones (no need to thaw them beforehand). If the sherbet becomes too hard, let it soften in the refrigerator for 30 minutes.

2 CUPS CHOPPED FRESH STRAWBERRIES

½ CUP SUGAR

2½ CUPS LOW-FAT BUTTERMILK

½ CUP HALF-AND-HALF

2 TEASPOONS LEMON JUICE

1 TEASPOON VANILLA EXTRACT

PINCH OF SALT

1. In a small bowl, combine 1 cup of strawberries and the sugar. Let it sit, stirring occasionally, until the sugar has begun to dissolve, about 10 minutes.
2. Transfer the strawberry mixture to a food processor or blender and process until smooth.
3. In a medium bowl, combine the buttermilk, half-and-half, lemon juice, vanilla, and salt.
4. Press the strawberry mixture through a fine-mesh sieve into the bowl. Stir, cover, and chill for at least 2 hours and up to 1 day.
5. Whisk the mixture and pour it into the canister of an ice-cream maker. Freeze according to the manufacturer's directions.
6. During last 5 minutes of freezing, add the remaining 1 cup of chopped strawberries.
7. Serve immediately or freeze the sherbet for a firmer consistency.

Almond-Lemon Cookies

MAKES 24 COOKIES

▸ CALORIES: 103, TOTAL FAT: 7 G, SATURATED FAT: 1 G, FIBER: 2 G,
SODIUM: 13 MG, CHOLESTEROL: 8 MG

Instead of using white flour, these cookies are made with finely ground blanched almonds. They are light and delicious—the perfect accompaniment to a cup of hot tea.

COOKING SPRAY
2 CUPS PLUS 24 WHOLE BLANCHED ALMONDS
⅔ CUP SUGAR
4 TEASPOONS GRATED LEMON ZEST
PINCH OF SALT
1 FREE-RANGE OR OMEGA-3 EGG
1 TEASPOON GROUND CINNAMON

1. Preheat the oven to 350°F.
2. Spray two baking sheets with cooking spray.
3. Place 2 cups of almonds in a food processor and process until finely ground.
4. Add the sugar, lemon zest, salt, and egg. Pulse ten times or until the dough forms a ball.
5. Shape the dough into balls using a tablespoonful of dough for each, making 24 balls.
6. Place the almond balls 1 inch apart on the baking sheets. Sprinkle them with cinnamon and press 1 whole almond into the center of each.
7. Bake the cookies for 16 minutes, or until the edges are golden brown.
8. Cool the cookies for 5 minutes in the pan; then remove them to a wire rack and let them cool completely before eating.

Carrot Cake Cookies

MAKES 30 COOKIES

▶ CALORIES: 83, TOTAL FAT: 6 G, SATURATED FAT: 3 G, FIBER: 1 G, SODIUM: 54 MG, CHOLESTEROL: 0 MG

This recipe delivers a divine slice of carrot cake that's just the right size. And see how easily you can make substitutions when baking: whole-wheat pastry flour replaces white flour, maple syrup replaces white sugar, and coconut oil replaces butter.

1 CUP WHOLE-WHEAT PASTRY FLOUR

1 TEASPOON BAKING POWDER

½ TEASPOON SALT

1 CUP ROLLED OATS

⅔ CUP CHOPPED WALNUTS

1 CUP PEELED, SHREDDED CARROTS

½ CUP MAPLE SYRUP, ROOM TEMPERATURE

½ CUP COCONUT OIL, WARMED UNTIL JUST MELTED

1 TEASPOON GRATED FRESH GINGER

1. Preheat the oven to 375°F.
2. Line two baking sheets with parchment paper.
3. In a large bowl, whisk together the flour, baking powder, salt, and oats. Add the walnuts and carrots.
4. In a small bowl, whisk together the maple syrup, coconut oil, and ginger.
5. Add the liquid ingredients to the flour mixture and stir until combined.
6. Drop the dough by the tablespoon onto the prepared baking sheets, leaving 2 inches between each.
7. Bake the cookies for 10 to 12 minutes, or until the cookies are golden brown.
8. Allow the cookies to cool before serving.

Peanut Butter Cups

MAKES 12 CUPS

▶ CALORIES: 220, TOTAL FAT: 14 G, SATURATED FAT: 6 G, FIBER: 2 G, SODIUM: 115 MG, CHOLESTEROL: 0 MG

Who doesn't love the combination of chocolate and peanut butter? These home-made versions of the checkout-line favorite are made with only five ingredients and have zero cholesterol.

2 SHEETS GRAHAM CRACKERS
¼ TEASPOON SALT
½ CUP PEANUT BUTTER
2 TABLESPOONS HONEY
12 OUNCES SEMISWEET CHOCOLATE, CHOPPED

1. Place 12 mini muffin cups in a 12-cup mini muffin pan.
2. In a food processor, process the graham crackers and salt until finely ground.
3. Transfer the graham cracker mix to a medium bowl and stir in the peanut butter and honey. Chill for 10 minutes.
4. Line a plate with plastic wrap. Make balls with 1 tablespoonful of peanut butter mixture until you have 12 balls. Flatten them slightly on the plate. Cover the peanut butter discs with plastic wrap and chill.
5. Place the chocolate in a bowl over simmering water and stir until smooth. Remove from the heat and let cool slightly.
6. Spoon 1 teaspoon of the chocolate into each mini muffin cup, spreading it so it covers the bottom and halfway up the sides. Chill for 30 minutes or until the chocolate hardens (keep the remaining chocolate at room temperature).
7. Press a peanut butter disk into each shell and spoon 1 tablespoon of the chocolate over the top. Chill until firm, about 1 hour.
8. Refrigerate the cups until you are ready to serve them.

Homemade Fudge Pops

MAKES 4 POPS

▶ CALORIES: 204, TOTAL FAT: 10 G, SATURATED FAT: 6 G, FIBER: 3 G, SODIUM: 50 MG, CHOLESTEROL: 6 MG

It's a lot easier than you think to create fudge pops yourself, and the bonus is you know exactly what's in them. You can find inexpensive popsicle molds in many different shapes in most stores where cookware is sold or online.

3½ OUNCES BITTERSWEET CHOCOLATE, CHOPPED
1 PACKET UNFLAVORED GELATIN
2 TABLESPOONS COLD WATER
1 CUP WHOLE MILK
2 TABLESPOONS SUGAR
1 TABLESPOON UNSWEETENED COCOA POWDER
1 TEASPOON VANILLA EXTRACT
¼ TEASPOON ALMOND EXTRACT

1. In a medium glass mixing bowl, place the chocolate and set aside.
2. In a small bowl, sprinkle the gelatin into the water and set aside.
3. Combine the milk, sugar, and cocoa powder in a small saucepan over medium heat. Whisk until the cocoa dissolves and the mixture comes to a simmer.
4. Remove the saucepan from the heat and pour the milk mixture over the chocolate. Let it stand for 2 minutes; then whisk the mixture until the chocolate is melted.
5. Whisk the vanilla extract, almond extract, and gelatin mixture into the chocolate.
6. Put ½ cup of the chocolate into four 4-ounce molds and freeze for at least 4 hours or overnight before serving.

Dark Chocolate Pudding

SERVES 6

▸ CALORIES: 190, TOTAL FAT: 11 G, SATURATED FAT: 2 G, FIBER: 7 G, SODIUM: 0 MG, CHOLESTEROL: 0 MG

Avocado in a dessert? Why not? The heart-healthful fat combines with dark cocoa and dates in this unique twist on chocolate pudding. The best part is you'd never know the secret ingredient from how it tastes.

2 AVOCADOS, PEELED AND PITTED

1 BANANA

½ CUP UNSWEETENED DARK COCOA POWDER

½ CUP DATES, PITTED, SOAKED IN WATER FOR
    A FEW HOURS, AND DRAINED

1 TEASPOON PURE VANILLA EXTRACT

1. In a food processor, combine all the ingredients. Purée until smooth, scraping the sides of the bowl as needed.
2. Chill the pudding for 3 to 4 hours before serving. The pudding may be served either out of a large bowl or in single-serving dishes.

Flourless Chocolate Cake

SERVES 16

▶ CALORIES: 159, TOTAL FAT: 12 G, SATURATED FAT: 9 G, FIBER: 2 G, SODIUM: 16 MG, CHOLESTEROL: 35 MG

Because this cake is made with unsweetened baking chocolate, the result isn't as sweet as you may be used to. If you find it too bitter, try using 70 percent dark chocolate instead. Serve it warm with a scoop of slow-churned vanilla ice cream on top.

½ CUP COCONUT OIL, PLUS FOR GREASING THE PAN

4 OUNCES UNSWEETENED BAKING CHOCOLATE

¼ CUP COCOA POWDER

¾ CUP HONEY

3 FREE-RANGE OR OMEGA-3 EGGS

1. Preheat the oven to 375°F.
2. Grease an 8-inch springform pan with coconut oil.
3. Fill the bottom pot of a double boiler with 1 to 2 inches of water and place the top pot over it (the water shouldn't touch the bottom of the top pot). Bring the water to a simmer and reduce the heat. Put the chocolate and coconut oil into the top pot and stir until melted and completely smooth.
4. In a medium bowl, combine the chocolate mixture with the cocoa powder, honey, and eggs, whisking briskly until smooth.
5. Pour the batter into the pan and bake for 20 to 25 minutes, or until the center holds firm when the pan is tilted slightly.
6. Cool the cake in the pan for 15 minutes; then carefully run a knife around the inner rim to loosen the cake. Remove the sides and let the cake cool completely before serving.

Resources

Cholesterol and Saturated Fat Levels in Foods

National Health Research Institutes. "Important Basics Food Charts: Cholesterol." *Asia Pacific Journal of Clinical Nutrition*. Accessed October 2013. http://apjcn. nhri.org.tw/server/info/books-phds/books/foodfacts/html/data/data2h.html.

Dietary Recommendations

21-Day Vegan Kickstart. "Resources: Your Kickstart Team." PCRM Physicians Committee for Responsible Medicine. Accessed October 2013. http://pcrm. org/kickstartHome/resources/bios.cfm.

Balch, James, and Jolie Root. *101 Amazing Healing Secrets*. Weiss Research Inc., 1998.

Beck, Leslie. "Fructose Can Trigger Cancer Cells to Grow Faster, Study Finds." *Globe and Mail*. Last modified November 30, 2010. http://www. theglobeandmail.com/life/health-and-fitness/fructose-can-trigger-cancer-cells-to-grow-faster-study-finds/article1316253/.

FDA (U.S. Food and Drug Administration). "Summary of Published Research on the Beneficial Effects of Fish Consumption and Omega-3 Fatty Acids for Certain Neurodevelopmental and Cardiovascular Endpoints: Section A—Cardiovascular Disease." Last modified January 15, 2013. http://www.fda.gov/ Food/FoodborneIllnessContaminants/Metals/ucm153053.htm.

HHS (U.S. Department of Health and Human Services.) *Your Guide to Lowering Your Blood Pressure with DASH*. Reprint. Bethesda, MD: National Institutes of Health, 2006. www.nhlbi.nih.gov/health/public/heart/hbp/dash/new_dash.pdf.

HHS (U.S. Department of Health and Human Services) and USDA (U.S. Drug Administration). "Dietary Guidelines for Americans 2005." Last modified May 1, 2008. www.health.gov/dietaryguidelines/dga2005/recommendations.htm.

Horizon Naturopathic. "Naturopathic Care Helps to Reduce Heart Disease Risk Factors." April 30, 2013. http://www.horizonnaturopathic.ca/naturo-pathic-care-helps-to-reduce-heart-disease-risk-factors/.

Klapper, Joseph Lee. *The Complete Idiot's Guide to Lowering Your Cholesterol.* New York: Alpha Books, 2006.

Livestrong.com. "Cholesterol." Accessed October 2013. www.livestrong.com/cholesterol/.

Livestrong.com "Nuts and Seeds." Accessed October 2013. www.livestrong.com/nuts-seeds/.

Lorna Vanderhaeghe Health Solutions, Inc. www.healthyimmunity.com.

Natural News. "Nutritional Deficiencies News, Articles and Information." Accessed October 2013. www.naturalnews.com/nutritional_deficiencies.html.

Pittman, Genevra. "Can Selenium Lower Cholesterol?" *Reuters.* May 16, 2011. www.reuters.com/article/2011/05/16/us-selenium-cholesterol-idUS-TRE74F80M20110516.

Root, Jolie. "The Extraordinary Benefits of Omega-3s." *Total Health Online.* Accessed October 2013. www.totalhealthmagazine.com/blog/Jolie-Root-LPN-LNC.html.

Whole Foods. Accessed October 2013. www.wholefoods.com.

World's Healthiest Foods. "What's New and Beneficial about Broccoli." Accessed November 19, 2013. http://www.whfoods.com/genpage.php?tname=foodspice&dbid=9.

Nutrition Labels

American Heart Association. "Reading Food Nutrition Labels." Last modified October 23, 2013. http://www.heart.org/HEARTORG/GettingHealthy/NutritionCenter/HeartSmartShopping/Reading-Food-Nutrition-Labels_UCM_300132_Article.jsp.

Plant Substances

Cleveland Clinic Foundation. "Plant Sterols and Stanols." Last modified July 15, 2009. http://my.clevelandclinic.org/healthy_living/cholesterol/hic_plant_sterols_and_stanols.aspx.

Additional Resources

American Heart Association. "Conditions: Cholesterol." Accessed 2013. www.heart.org/HEARTORG/Conditions/Cholesterol/Cholesterol_UCM_001089_SubHomePage.jsp.

American Heart Association. "Cooking for Lower Cholesterol." Last modified September 6, 2013. www.heart.org/HEARTORG/Conditions/Cholesterol/PreventionTreatmentofHighCholesterol/Cooking-for-Lower-Cholesterol_UCM_305630_Article.jsp.

CDC (Centers for Disease Control and Prevention) and National Center for Health Statistics. "Cholesterol." Last modified May 30, 2013. www.cdc.gov/nchs/fastats/cholest.htm.

FDA (U.S. Food and Drug Administration). "Controlling Cholesterol with Statins." FDA Consumer Health Information. Last modified August 20, 2013. www.fda.gov/ForConsumers/ConsumerUpdates/ucm048496.htm.

Houston, Mark C. *What Your Doctor May Not Tell You About Heart Disease.* New York: Grand Central Life & Style, 2012.

Mann, Denise. "Proper Nutrition and Heart Health: WebMD's Top 5 Vitamins and Minerals for Heart Health. Part 2 of a Three-Part Series." WebMD. Accessed October 2013. http://www.webmd.com/heart-disease/features/diet-lowers-high-cholesterol.

National Cholesterol Education Program. *Third Report of the Expert Panel on Detection, Evaluation, and Treatment of High Blood Cholesterol in Adults (Adult Treatment Panel III).* National Institutes of Health. September 2002. www.nhlbi. nih.gov/guidelines/cholesterol.

National Cholesterol Education Program. "High Blood Cholesterol: What You Need to Know." National Institutes of Health. Last modified June 2005. www. nhlbi.nih.gov/health/public/heart/chol/wyntk.htm#numbers.

National Research Council. *Dietary Reference Intakes for Energy, Carbohydrate, Fiber, Fat, Fatty Acids, Cholesterol, Protein, and Amino Acids (Macronutrients).* Washington, DC: National Academies Press, 2005.

Index

Made in the USA
Lexington, KY
02 December 2014